Therapeutic Ultrasound in Dentistry

Tarek El-Bialy • Eiji Tanaka •
Dror Aizenbud

Editors

Therapeutic Ultrasound in Dentistry

Applications for Dentofacial Repair, Regeneration, and Tissue Engineering

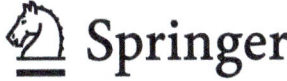 Springer

Editors
Tarek El-Bialy
Dentistry/Orthodontics and Biomedical
Engineering
University of Alberta
Edmonton, Alberta, Canada

Eiji Tanaka
Department of Orthodontics and
Dentofacial Orthopedics
Institute of Biomedical Sciences
Tokushima University Graduate School
Tokushima, Japan

Dror Aizenbud
Technion—Faculty of Medicine
Oral Biology Research Laboratory
Rambam Health Care Campus
Haifa, Israel

ISBN 978-3-030-09769-1   ISBN 978-3-319-66323-4   (eBook)
https://doi.org/10.1007/978-3-319-66323-4

Printed on acid-free paper

This Springer imprint is published by the registered company Springer International Publishing AG part of Springer Nature.
The registered company address is: Gewerbestrasse 11, 6330 Cham, Switzerland

Contents

Acoustic Description and Mechanical Action of Low-Intensity Pulsed Ultrasound (LIPUS)

1

Tarek El-Bialy and Harmanpreet Kaur

Abstract

Ultrasound is a mechanical wave that can pass through media and tissues. Because ultrasound is a mechanical wave, the stress produced by these waves can produce different cellular and tissue stimulations at the cellular and subcellular levels. Although the exact fine details of these stresses on the cellular/subcellular levels have not been fully understood, this chapter sheds light on the current information/literature that has been studying both mechanical and nature of these waves and their interaction with living tissues.

diagnostic, and operative tool [1, 2]. Some therapeutic ultrasound and some operative ultrasound use intensities as high as $1–3$ W/cm^2 and can result in considerable heating of the living tissues. Other types of ultrasound are called low-intensity ultrasound with frequencies around $30–150$ mW/cm^2. Therapeutic ultrasound is widely used, mainly in sports medicine and myofunctional therapy; in the reduction of joint stiffness, muscle pain, and spasms; and in improving muscle mobility [3]. Also, therapeutic ultrasound can become a powerful non-viral method for the delivery of genes into cells and tissues [4, 5].

1.1 Acoustic Description of Low-Intensity Pulsed Ultrasound

Ultrasound is an acoustic pressure wave at frequencies that are above the human hearing frequency limit. Ultrasound wave is transmitted into and through biological tissues and hence produces different metabolic activities. Ultrasound has been widely used in medicine as a therapeutic,

1.2 Mechanical Action

In the field of medicine, ultrasound is classified according to its waveform: continuous and pulsed (Fig. 1.1), or on the basis of its application: diagnostic, operative, and therapeutic [6].

Low-intensity pulsed ultrasound (LIPUS) is a form of an acoustic wave that produces micromechanical strain in the tissue through which it passes, leading to biochemical events [7, 8]. It is a safe, easy to use, and cost-effective method to facilitate the healing of non-healing fractured bone and it has been approved by the US Food and Drug Administration (FDA) [9]. It has been used to enhance bone regeneration and healing as well as reduces treatment time after

T. El-Bialy (✉)
Dentistry/Orthodontics and Biomedical Engineering, University of Alberta, Edmonton, Alberta, Canada
e-mail: telbialy@ualberta.ca

H. Kaur
Department of Dentistry, University of Alberta, Edmonton, AB, Canada

© Springer International Publishing AG, part of Springer Nature 2018
T. El-Bialy et al. (eds.), *Therapeutic Ultrasound in Dentistry*,
https://doi.org/10.1007/978-3-319-66323-4_1

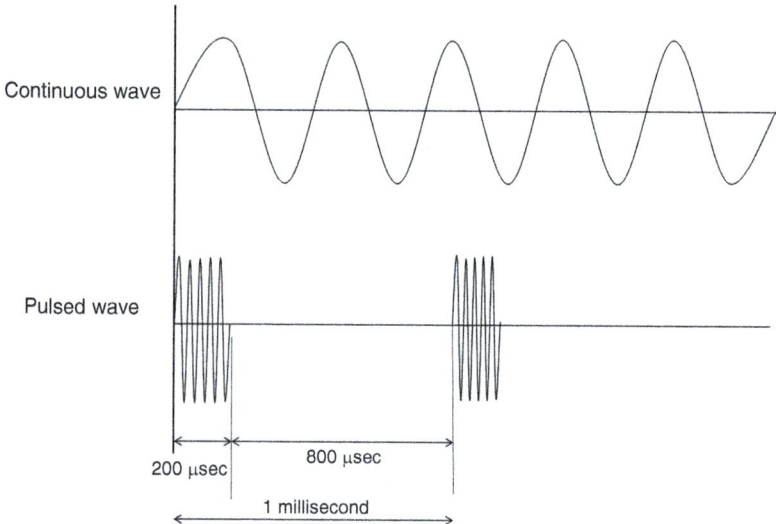

Fig. 1.1 Ultrasound waveform: continuous and pulsed

Continuous wave

Pulsed wave

200 μsec

800 μsec

1 millisecond

distraction osteogenesis [10]. LIPUS also stimulates new blood vessel formation and hence enhances endochondral bone formation [11, 12]. In vitro studies have shown to increase cell count in fibroblast and osteoblast cell culture [13, 14] with increased transforming growth factor β1 (TGF-β1) expression; decreased Interleukin-6 (IL-6) and tumor necrosis factor-α (TNF-α) expression [15]; and increased Runt related transcription factor 2 (RUNX2), alkaline phosphatase (ALP), vascular endothelial growth factor (VEGF), osteocalcin (OCN), and bone morphogenetic protein-2 (BMP-2) expression [16–19]. Similar results were seen in bone marrow-derived stem cells and animal studies. Increased aggrecan (ACAN) and collagen II (Col II) expression has been supported in several studies [20–24].

The exact mechanism of LIPUS effects on biological tissues is still not completely understood. The biophysical effects of ultrasound are mostly studied in the in vitro studies, and these results are extrapolated to the in vivo studies. Since different studies use different ultrasound parameters and various experimental setups, it is very difficult to completely understand the mechanism of action. The potential biological response of therapeutic ultrasound can be divided into thermal and nonthermal effects.

Therapeutic ultrasound produces vibrational forces as it passes through the cell culture or the tissue. These vibrational forces cause a rise in temperature due to absorption of the energy. Heat generation is dependent on the intensity applied and the waveform. Pulsed ultrasound causes lower heat generation as compared to continuous waveform. Lehman et al. [25] showed a rise in temperature to 41 °C after 1 min and to 44 °C after 3 min when 1 MHz continuous ultrasound was applied. However, in a recent study by Xue et al. [26], pulsed ultrasound also showed increase in temperature of about 3 °C after 20 min. These temperature variations can affect thermo-sensitive enzymes like matrix metalloproteinase. Increase in temperature of 2 °C resulted in three times fold change in reaction rate for bone matrix remodeling [27]. The amount of energy absorbed is dependent on the tissue density, making bone responsive to heat. This effect is considered useful in physiotherapy where ultrasound is used for muscle stiffness. Thermal effect of ultrasound also includes increased blood flow, decreased muscle pain and spasm, and increased collagen extensibility.

LIPUS produces a nonthermal effect which causes cavitation and micro-streaming and affects the cell membrane. Cavitation is the growth and oscillation of gaseous cavities which grow rapidly and collapse leading to change in the cell membrane. These changes increase the cell membrane permeability and hence increase the cellular uptake of the extracellular ions, growth factors, and drugs [28]. But when the bubble grows in size so that it collapses, it results in permanent membrane damage and cell death; this is known as unstable cavitation [29]. Acoustic streaming is the circular movement of the fluid around the vibrating structures like the cell membranes or the oscillating gas bubbles. These movements produce stress on the structures leading to the formation of pores for a short period of time. The increase in the membrane permeability and movement of fluid around it causes the delivery of the therapeutic agents into the cell [30]. However, the intensity of LIPUS is too low to induce cavitation or cell membrane destruction [31]. The mechanical energy of LIPUS when applied to biological tissues or cells induces strain on the cell membrane affecting the mechanosensitive elements [32]. In "bilayer sonophore model" proposed by Krasovitski et al. [33], it explains the changes in cell membrane bilayer with ultrasound application. In positive pressure, the cell membrane layers are pushed together, while in negative pressure, the membranes are pulled apart. These movements also cause the activation of mechanosensitive elements. The process by which cell senses the mechanical load and transduces it into a cascade of cellular and molecular events is called mechanotransduction. Mechanosensitive elements, including cytoskeleton, stretch-activated ion channels, integrins, and G-protein receptors, have been extensively explained in the literature.

1.3 Mechanotransduction and LIPUS

Microfilaments, microtubules, and intermediate filaments like actin, talin, vinculin, and filamin A are the structural units of the cytoskeleton that maintain the cellular shape during the application of mechanical load. The cytoskeleton components provide a direct link between the adhesion receptors and the nucleus. Integrins and cadherins are coupled with cytoskeleton filament on one end and nuclear scaffold, nucleoli, chromatin, or DNA in the nucleus on the other end [34]. When the mechanical load is applied, cytoskeleton filaments bear the impact and reorganize themselves and activate the biochemical events that influence cell survival and protein synthesis in addition to spreading and migration [35]. Many studies have shown activation of signal transduction and gene expression with alteration in cytoskeleton structure [36–38]. Previous studies have shown increased polymerization of actin filament and activation of integrin with ultrasound application [39–41].

Stretch-activated ion channels (SAC) play an important role not only in maintaining the resting membrane potential but also in cell volume. Upon activation, these channels allow movement of ions like Na^+, Ca^{2+}, and K^+ in or out of the cells. Na^+ ion first enters the cells causing depolarization of the membrane which is followed by Ca^{2+} entry [42]. Ca^{2+} ion concentration in the cell also increases due to the release of ions from intracellular reservoirs: endoplasmic reticulum, sarcoplasmic reticulum, and mitochondria. Increased Ca^{2+} ions after mechanical stimulation are seen in different cell types including smooth muscle cells, fibroblasts, osteoblasts, and chondrocytes. SAC after mechanical loading causes phosphorylation of focal adhesion kinase (FAK) and paxillin [43], aggrecan gene expression, and cell proliferation [44, 45]. LIPUS has also shown increased Ca^{2+} ion concentration causing proteoglycan synthesis in chondrocytes, and this effect was abolished by inhibiting Ca^{2+} ions [21].

Integrins are transmembrane glycoprotein receptors composed of two subunits: α and β. Their primary function is the attachment of the cell to its extracellular matrix (ECM). The combination of α and β subunits is specific for the cell type and determines the ligand specificity. α5β1 is a fibronectin-specific integrin present in chondrocytes. Integrin signaling across the cell membrane can be "inside out" where the binding of integrin to its ECM components is regulated by the inside of the cell, or it can be "outside in"; i.e., integrin binding to ECM component leads to biochemical events in the cell [46]. The structure of integrin has three domains: extracellular domain, membrane-spanning region, and a cytoplasmic tail. At resting stage, the extracellular domain has "bent" conformation. When the mechanical load is applied, this changes to "upright" structure exposing the binding sites to ECM [47]. The cytoplasmic tail end activates FAK and further recruits talin and paxillin which are cytoplasmic proteins. These proteins are triggered to form large multi-protein complex called focal adhesion molecule during integrin activation. This further leads to activation and organization of either cytoskeleton component of the cell [48, 49]. Studies have shown that mechanical stresses produced by LIPUS have led to increase in gene expression and protein synthesis in chondrocytes and osteoblasts via integrin activation [50–52]. Many studies in the literature have shown that ultrasound exposure augments membrane expression of integrins [50, 53] and hence results in reorganization of cytoskeleton and maturation of osteoblasts [41] and chondrogenic differentiation of human mesenchymal stem cell [54]. Mechanical loading by LIPUS has shown to increase phosphorylation of focal adhesion molecule like FAK and Src which are downstream regulators of MAPK signaling pathway [55–57].

Mitogen-activated protein kinases (MAPKs) are serine-threonine protein kinases that are extensively studied in many cell types, especially in osteoblast and chondrocyte. These protein kinases respond to the external stimuli and regulate the cellular events by affecting the gene and protein expression in various cellular processes like cell growth, differentiation, survival, and cell death. These include extracellular signal-regulated kinase1/2 (ERK1/2), c-Jun N-terminal kinase (JNK), and p38 kinase. ERK1/2 is preferentially activated in response to growth factors, while JNK and p38 kinase are more responsive to stress stimuli. In osteoblast, MAPKs regulate bone mass by acting as a mediator in osteoblast differentiation. There is an increase in activator protein-1 (AP-1), a transcription factor for osteoblast differentiation, with MAPK activation [58]. In chondrocytes, JNK plays a minor role,

while ERK1/2 and p38 are important for chondrogenesis [59]. Activated MAPK further phosphorylates various intracellular factors involved in cellular metabolism including membrane transporters, cytoskeletal elements, and transcription factors [60]. Studies on LIPUS have shown increased phosphorylation of ERK1/2 and p38 in osteoblasts and chondrocytes [57, 61–65]. Activation of MAPK employs core three-kinase cascade consisting of MAP 3K which phosphorylates and activates MAP 2K which then phosphorylates and increases the activity of MAPK. Dephosphorylation of MAPK by phosphatase is an important negative control.

In conclusion, the mechanical vibration that LIPUS produces activates the cell membrane cascade which then transfers to the cell nucleus. In most cases, these mechanical stimulations upregulate an array of genes in the cell nucleus that enhances matrix formation and cell viability as well as cell multiplication.

References

1. Dyson M. Therapeutic applications of ultrasound. In: Nyborg WL, Ziskin MC, editors. Biological effects of ultrasound. New York: Churchill Livingstone; 1985. p. 121–33.
2. Ziskin M. Applications of ultrasound in medicine-comparison with other modalities. In: Repacholi MH, Grandolfo M, Rindi A, editors. Ultrasound: medical applications, biological effects, and hazard potential. New York: Plenum Press; 1987. p. 49–59.
3. Graber TM. The clinical implications of unique metabolic processes in the human TMJ. In: Sachdeva R, editor. Orthodontics for the next millennium. Dallas, TX: Baylor University Press; 1997.
4. Duvshani-Eshet M, Adam D, Machluf M. The effects of albumin-coated microbubbles in DNA delivery mediated by therapeutic ultrasound. J Control Release. 2006a;112:156–66.
5. Duvshani-Eshet M, Baruch L, Kesselman E, Shimoni E, Machluf M. Therapeutic ultrasound-mediated DNA to cell and nucleus: bioeffects revealed by confocal and atomic force microscopy. Gene Ther. 2006b;13:163–72.
6. Kasturi G, Adler RA. Mechanical means to improve bone strength: ultrasound and vibration. Curr Rheumatol Rep. 2011;13(3):251–6. https://doi.org/10.1007/s11926-011-0177-7

7. Tanaka E, Kuroda S, Horiuchi S, Tabata A, El-Bialy T. Low-intensity pulsed ultrasound in dentofacial tissue engineering. Ann Biomed Eng. 2015;43(4):871–86. https://doi.org/10.1007/s10439-015-1274-y

8. Claes L, Willie B. The enhancement of bone regeneration by ultrasound. Prog Biophys Mol Biol. 2007;93 (1–3):384–98. https://doi.org/10.1016/j.pbiomolbio. 2006.07.021

9. Bashardoust Tajali S, Houghton P, MacDermid JC, Grewal R. Effects of low-intensity pulsed ultrasound therapy on fracture healing: a systematic review and meta-analysis. Am J Phys Med Rehabil. 2012;91 (4):349–67. https://doi.org/10.1097/PHM. 0b013e31822419ba

10. El-Bialy TH, Elgazzar RF, Megahed EE, Royston TJ. Effects of ultrasound modes on mandibular osteodistraction. J Dent Res. 2008;87(10):953–7.

11. Shimazaki A, Inui K, Azuma Y, Nishimura N, Yamano Y. Low-intensity pulsed ultrasound accelerates bone maturation in distraction osteogenesis in rabbits. J Bone Joint Surg Br. 2000;82(7):1077–82.

12. Katano M, Naruse K, Uchida K, Mikuni-Takagaki Y, Takaso M, Itoman M, Urabe K. Low intensity pulsed ultrasound accelerates delayed healing process by reducing the time required for the completion of endochondral ossification in the aged mouse femur fracture model. Exp Anim. 2011;60(4):385–95.

13. Doan N, Reher P, Meghji S, Harris M. In vitro effects of therapeutic ultrasound on cell proliferation, protein synthesis, and cytokine production by human fibroblasts, osteoblasts, and monocytes. J Oral Maxillofac Surg. 1999;57(4):409–19. discussion 420

14. Sun JS, Hong RC, Chang WH, Chen LT, Lin FH, Liu HC. In vitro effects of low-intensity ultrasound stimulation on the bone cells. J Biomed Mater Res. 2001;57 (3):449–56.

15. Li JK, Chang WH, Lin JC, Ruaan RC, Liu HC, Sun JS. Cytokine release from osteoblasts in response to ultrasound stimulation. Biomaterials. 2003;24 (13):2379–85. https://doi.org/10.1016/S0142-9612(03)00033-4

16. Naruse K, Sekiya H, Harada Y, Iwabuchi S, Kozai Y, Kawamata R, Kashima I, et al. Prolonged endochondral bone healing in senescence is shortened by low-intensity pulsed ultrasound in a manner dependent on COX-2. Ultrasound Med Biol. 2010;36 (7):1098–108. https://doi.org/10.1016/j.ultrasmedbio. 2010.04.011

17. Naruse K, Miyauchi A, Itoman M, Mikuni-Takagaki Y. Distinct anabolic response of osteoblast to low-intensity pulsed ultrasound. J Bone Miner Res. 2003;18(2):360–9. https://doi.org/10.1359/jbmr.2003. 18.2.360

18. Ikeda K, Takayama T, Suzuki N, Shimada K, Otsuka K, Ito K. Effects of low-intensity pulsed ultrasound on the differentiation of C2C12 cells. Life Sci. 2006;79(20):1936–43. https://doi.org/10.1016/j.lfs. 2006.06.029

19. Takayama T, Suzuki N, Ikeda K, Shimada T, Suzuki A, Maeno M, Otsuka K, Ito K. Low-intensity pulsed ultrasound stimulates osteogenic differentiation in ROS 17/2.8 cells. Life Sci. 2007;80(10):965–71. https://doi.org/10.1016/j.lfs.2006.11.037

20. Parvizi J, Wu CC, Lewallen DG, Greenleaf JF, Bolander ME. Low-intensity ultrasound stimulates proteoglycan synthesis in rat chondrocytes by increasing aggrecan gene expression. J Orthop Res. 1999;17 (4):488–94. https://doi.org/10.1002/jor.1100170405

21. Parvizi J, Parpura V, Greenleaf JF, Bolander ME. Calcium signaling is required for ultrasound-stimulated aggrecan synthesis by rat chondrocytes. J Orthop Res. 2002;20(1):51–7. https://doi.org/10.1016/ S0736-0266(01)00069-9

22. Mukai S, Ito H, Nakagawa Y, Akiyama H, Miyamoto M, Nakamura T. Transforming growth factor-beta1 mediates the effects of low-intensity pulsed ultrasound in chondrocytes. Ultrasound Med Biol. 2005;31(12):1713–21. https://doi.org/10.1016/j. ultrasmedbio.2005.07.012

23. Zhang Z-J, Huckle J, Francomano CA, Spencer RGS. The effects of pulsed low-intensity ultrasound on chondrocyte viability, proliferation, gene expression and matrix production. Ultrasound Med Biol. 2003;29(11):1645–51.

24. Zhang Z, Huckle J, Francomano CA, Spencer RGS. The influence of pulsed low-intensity ultrasound on matrix production of chondrocytes at different stages of differentiation: an explant study. Ultrasound Med Biol. 2002;28(11–12):1547–53.

25. Lehmann JF, Mcmillan JA, Brunner GD, Blumberg JB. Comparative study of the efficiency of short-wave, microwave and ultrasonic diathermy in heating the hip joint. Arch Phys Med Rehabil. 1959;40 (December):510–2.

26. Xue H, Zheng J, Cui Z, Bai X, Li G, Zhang C, He S, et al. Low-intensity pulsed ultrasound accelerates tooth movement via activation of the BMP-2 signaling pathway. PloS One. 2013;8(7):e68926. https://doi.org/10. 1371/journal.pone.0068926

27. Kusano K, Miyaura C, Inada M, Tamura T, Ito A, Nagase H, Kamoi K, Suda T. Regulation of matrix metalloproteinases (MMP-2, -3, -9, and -13) by interleukin-1 and interleukin-6 in mouse calvaria: association of MMP induction with bone resorption. Endocrinology. 1998;139(3):1338–45. https://doi.org/ 10.1210/endo.139.3.5818

28. Mitragotri S. Healing sound: the use of ultrasound in drug delivery and other therapeutic applications. Nat Rev Drug Discov. 2005;4(3):255–60. https://doi.org/ 10.1038/nrd1662

29. Dyson M. Non-thermal cellular effects of ultrasound. Br J Cancer Suppl. 1982;5(March):165–71.

30. Frenkel V. Ultrasound mediated delivery of drugs and genes to solid tumors. Adv Drug Deliv Rev. 2008;60 (10):1193–208. https://doi.org/10.1016/j.addr.2008. 03.007

31. Padilla F, Puts R, Vico L, Raum K. Stimulation of bone repair with ultrasound: a review of the possible mechanic effects. Ultrasonics. 2014;54(5):1125–45. https://doi.org/10.1016/j.ultras.2014.01.004

32. Sarvazyan A. Diversity of biomedical applications of acoustic radiation force. Ultrasonics. 2010;50(2):230–4. https://doi.org/10.1016/j.ultras.2009.10.001

33. Krasovitski B, Frenkel V, Shoham S, Kimmel E. Intramembrane cavitation as a unifying mechanism for ultrasound-induced bioeffects. Proc Natl Acad Sci U S A. 2011;108(8):3258–63. https://doi.org/10.1073/pnas.1015771108

34. Wang N, Tytell JD, Ingber DE. Mechanotransduction at a distance: mechanically coupling the extracellular matrix with the nucleus. Nat Rev Mol Cell Biol. 2009;10(1):75–82. https://doi.org/10.1038/nrm2594

35. Wang JH-C, Thampatty BP. An introductory review of cell mechanobiology. Biomech Model Mechanobiol. 2006;5(1):1–16. https://doi.org/10.1007/s10237-005-0012-z

36. Schmidt CE, Horwitz AF, Lauffenburger DA, Sheetz MP. Integrin-cytoskeletal interactions in migrating fibroblasts are dynamic, asymmetric, and regulated. J Cell Biol. 1993;123(4):977–91.

37. Wang N, Butler JP, Ingber DE. Mechanotransduction across the cell surface and through the cytoskeleton. Science. 1993;260(5111):1124–7.

38. Urbich C, Dernbach E, Reissner A, Vasa M, Zeiher AM, Dimmeler S. Shear stress-induced endothelial cell migration involves integrin signaling via the fibronectin receptor subunits alpha(5) and beta(1). Arterioscler Thromb Vasc Biol. 2002;22(1):69–75.

39. Juffermans LJ, van Dijk A, Jongenelen CAM, Drukarch B, Reijerkerk A, de Vries HE, Kamp O, Musters RJP. Ultrasound and microbubble-induced intra- and intercellular bioeffects in primary endothelial cells. Ultrasound Med Biol. 2009;35(11):1917–27. https://doi.org/10.1016/j.ultrasmedbio.2009.06.1091

40. Uddin SMZ, Hadjiargyrou M, Cheng J, Zhang S, Minyi H, Qin Y-X. Reversal of the detrimental effects of simulated microgravity on human osteoblasts by modified low intensity pulsed ultrasound. Ultrasound Med Biol. 2013;39(5):804–12. https://doi.org/10.1016/j.ultrasmedbio.2012.11.016

41. Yang R-S, Lin W-L, Chen Y-Z, Tang C-H, Huang T-H, Bing-Yuh L, Wen-Mei F. Regulation by ultrasound treatment on the integrin expression and differentiation of osteoblasts. Bone. 2005;36(2):276–83. https://doi.org/10.1016/j.bone.2004.10.009

42. Guilak F. The deformation behavior and viscoelastic properties of chondrocytes in articular cartilage. Biorheology. 2000;37(1–2):27–44.

43. Lee HS, Millward-Sadler SJ, Wright MO, Nuki G, Salter DM. Integrin and mechanosensitive ion channel-dependent tyrosine phosphorylation of focal adhesion proteins and beta-catenin in human articular chondrocytes after mechanical stimulation. J Bone Mineral Res Off J Am Soc Bone Mineral Res. 2000;15(8):1501–9. https://doi.org/10.1359/jbmr.2000.15.8.1501

44. Salter DM, Millward-Sadler SJ, Nuki G, Wright MO. Differential responses of chondrocytes from normal and osteoarthritic human articular cartilage to mechanical stimulation. Biorheology. 2002;39 (1–2):97–108.

45. Wu QQ, Chen Q. Mechanoregulation of chondrocyte proliferation, maturation, and hypertrophy: ion-channel dependent transduction of matrix deformation signals. Exp Cell Res. 2000;256(2):383–91. https://doi.org/10.1006/excr.2000.4847

46. Giancotti FG, Ruoslahti E. Integrin signaling. Science. 1999;285(5430):1028–32.

47. Campbell ID, Humphries MJ. Integrin structure, activation, and interactions. Cold Spring Harb Perspect Biol. 2011;3(3). https://doi.org/10.1101/cshperspect.a004994

48. Kuo J-C, Han X, Hsiao C-T, Yates JR, Waterman CM. Analysis of the Myosin-II-responsive focal adhesion proteome reveals a role for β-Pix in negative regulation of focal adhesion maturation. Nat Cell Biol. 2011;13(4):383–93. https://doi.org/10.1038/ncb2216

49. Schiller HB, Friedel CC, Boulegue C, Fässler R. Quantitative proteomics of the integrin adhesome show a myosin II-dependent recruitment of LIM domain proteins. EMBO Rep. 2011;12(3):259–66. https://doi.org/10.1038/embor.2011.5

50. Whitney NP, Lamb AC, Louw TM, Subramanian A. Integrin-mediated mechanotransduction pathway of low-intensity continuous ultrasound in human chondrocytes. Ultrasound Med Biol. 2012;38 (10):1734–43. https://doi.org/10.1016/j.ultrasmedbio.2012.06.002

51. Watabe H, Furuhama T, Tani-Ishii N, Mikuni-Takagaki Y. Mechanotransduction activates $A_5\beta_1$ integrin and PI3K/Akt signaling pathways in mandibular osteoblasts. Exp Cell Res. 2011;317(18):2642–9. https://doi.org/10.1016/j.yexcr.2011.07.015

52. Iwabuchi Y, Tanimoto K, Tanne Y, Inubushi T, Kamiya T, Kunimatsu R, Hirose N, et al. Effects of low-intensity pulsed ultrasound on the expression of cyclooxygenase-2 in mandibular condylar chondrocytes. J Oral Facial Pain Headache. 2014;28 (3):261–8.

53. Lee D-Y, Yeh C-R, Chang S-F, Lee P-L, Chien S, Cheng C-K, Chiu J-J. Integrin-mediated expression of bone formation-related genes in osteoblast-like cells in response to fluid shear stress: roles of extracellular matrix, Shc, and mitogen-activated protein kinase. J Bone Miner Res Off J Am Soc Bone Miner Res. 2008;23(7):1140–9. https://doi.org/10.1359/jbmr.080302

54. Schumann D, Kujat R, Zellner J, Angele MK, Nerlich M, Mayr E, Angele P. Treatment of human mesenchymal stem cells with pulsed low intensity ultrasound enhances the chondrogenic phenotype in vitro. Biorheology. 2006;43(3–4):431–43.

55. Cheng K, Xia P, Lin Q, Shen S, Gao M, Ren S, Li X. Effects of low-intensity pulsed ultrasound on integrin-FAK-PI3K/Akt mechanochemical transduction

in rabbit osteoarthritis chondrocytes. Ultrasound Med Biol. 2014;40(7):1609–18. https://doi.org/10.1016/j.ultrasmedbio.2014.03.002

56. Barberis L, Wary KK, Fiucci G, Liu F, Hirsch E, Brancaccio M, Altruda F, Tarone G, Giancotti FG. Distinct roles of the adaptor protein Shc and focal adhesion kinase in integrin signaling to ERK. J Biol Chem. 2000;275(47):36532–40. https://doi.org/10.1074/jbc.M002487200

57. Choi BH, Choi MH, Kwak M-G, Min B-H, Woo ZH, Park SR. Mechanotransduction pathways of low-intensity ultrasound in C-28/I2 human chondrocyte cell line. Proc Inst Mech Eng H J Eng Med. 2007;221(5):527–35.

58. Greenblatt MB, Shim J-H, Glimcher LH. Mitogen-activated protein kinase pathways in osteoblasts. Ann Rev Cell Dev Biol. 2013;29(1):63–79. https://doi.org/10.1146/annurev-cellbio-101512-122347

59. Stanton L-A, Michael Underhill T, Beier F. MAP kinases in chondrocyte differentiation. Develop Biol. 2003;263(2):165–75.

60. Kyriakis JM, Avruch J. Mammalian MAPK signal transduction pathways activated by stress and inflammation: a 10-year update. Physiological Reviews. 2012;92(2):689–737. https://doi.org/10.1152/physrev.00028.2011

61. Li X, Li J, Cheng K, Lin Q, Wang D, Zhang H, An H, Gao M, Chen A. Effect of low-intensity pulsed ultrasound on MMP-13 and MAPKs signaling pathway in rabbit knee osteoarthritis. Cell Biochem Biophys. 2011;61(2):427–34. https://doi.org/10.1007/s12013-011-9206-4

62. Ren L, Yang Z, Song J, Wang Z, Deng F, Li W. Involvement of p38 MAPK pathway in low intensity pulsed ultrasound induced osteogenic differentiation of human periodontal ligament cells. Ultrasonics. 2012;53(3):686–90. https://doi.org/10.1016/j.ultras.2012.10.008

63. Sato M, Nagata K, Kuroda S, Horiuchi S, Nakamura T, Karima M, Inubushi T, Tanaka E. Low-intensity pulsed ultrasound activates integrin-mediated mechanotransduction pathway in synovial cells. Ann Biomed Eng. 2014;42(10):2156–63. https://doi.org/10.1007/s10439-014-1081-x

64. Xia P, Ren S, Lin Q, Cheng K, Shen S, Gao M, Li X. Low-intensity pulsed ultrasound affects chondrocyte extracellular matrix production via an integrin-mediated p38 MAPK signaling pathway. Ultrasound Med Biol. 2015;41(6):1690–700. https://doi.org/10.1016/j.ultrasmedbio.2015.01.014

65. Chen M-H, Sun J-S, Liao S-Y, Tai P-A, Li T-C, Chen M-H. Low-intensity pulsed ultrasound stimulates matrix metabolism of human annulus fibrosus cells mediated by transforming growth factor β1 and extracellular signal-regulated kinase pathway. Connect Tissue Res. 2015;56(3):219–27. https://doi.org/10.3109/03008207.2015.1016609

Mechanisms of LIPUS on Dentofacial Bioengineering

Natsuko Tanabe, Akihiro Yasue, and Eiji Tanaka

Abstract

LIPUS has been used by various people who have bone fracture as the instrument of treatment. However, the mechanism of LIPUS has been still elusive. In this chapter, the biological mechanism of LIPUS is described. Furthermore, in oral and maxillofacial region, structures of tissues and organs are very unique and complex in their development and function. This complexity makes difficult for their tissue engineering. Interestingly, mostly dentofacial diseases are implicated by inflammation. In this chapter, cellular or molecular biological mechanism of LIPUS, biological problems in dentofacial bioengineering, and also possibilities of dentofacial bioengineering and anti-inflammatory effects are discussed.

N. Tanabe (✉)
Department of Biochemistry, Nihon University School of Dentistry, Tokyo, Japan
e-mail: tanabe.natsuko@nihon-u.ac.jp

A. Yasue
Department of Orthodontics and Dentofacial Orthopedics, Institute of Biomedical Sciences, Tokushima University Graduate School, Tokushima, Japan

E. Tanaka
Department of Orthodontics and Dentofacial Orthopedics, Institute of Biomedical Sciences, Tokushima University Graduate School, Tokushima, Japan

Department of Orthodontics, King Abdulaziz University, Jeddah, Saudi Arabia

2.1 Cellular or Molecular Biological Mechanism of LIPUS

LIPUS exerts a variety of direct and indirect effects such as acoustic radiation force, acoustic streaming, and propagation of surface waves, thus promoting fluid flow-induced circulation and redistribution of nutrients, oxygen, and signaling molecules. In addition, the transformation of acoustic wave energy into heat can be ignored, and cavitation at the pressure levels delivered by LIPUS normally does not occur. Previous studies have reported that LIPUS promotes osteoblast differentiation and osteogenesis in vitro. These reports indicate that cells constituting dentofacial area respond to mechanical stimulation of LIPUS. These reports indicate that cells constituting maxillofacial area have biologic response to mechanical stimulation of LIPUS.

The greater than 200 mW/cm^2 intensity LIPUS caused cell death, whereas the smaller than 120 mW/cm^2 retained >95% cell viability in chondrocyte [1]. LIPUS is usually performed with an intensity of 30 mW/cm^2 SATA, 1.5 MHz, 1 kHz, pulsed with an exposure time of 20 min per day for clinical studies. Previous studies have reported that LIPUS promotes osteoblast differentiation and osteogenesis in vitro [2–4]. LIPUS also suppresses LPS-induced inflammatory chemokines in osteoblasts [5].

Particularly, the biological responses of LIPUS involve mechanosensitive receptors such as ion

© Springer International Publishing AG, part of Springer Nature 2018
T. El-Bialy et al. (eds.), *Therapeutic Ultrasound in Dentistry*,
https://doi.org/10.1007/978-3-319-66323-4_2

channels, integrins, G protein-coupled receptors, and P2 receptors [3, 6, 7]. It has been postulated that LIPUS may transmit signals into the cell through an integrin that may act as a mechanoreceptor on the cell membrane [6]. The attachment of various focal adhesion adaptor proteins is stimulated when the signals of LIPUS are transmitted to integrin molecules. LIPUS also phosphorylated focal adhesion kinase (FAK). LIPUS induces upregulation of phosphorylated FAK in the synovial cells. FAK phosphorylation inhibition also led to significant downregulation of mitogen-activated protein kinase (MAPK) phosphorylation. In addition, LIPUS affects the the activation of integrins including the downstream of signaling pathway on human skin fibroblasts *in vitro*. Integrins act as a link between extracellular matrix, cytoskeletal proteins, and actin filaments. Treatment with anti-integrin b1 and b3 antibodies or transfection with siRNA against integrin b1 and b3 showed inhibitory effect on cyclooxygenase (COX)-2expression. Furthermore, LIPUS treatment to cementoblasts stimulates cell metabolism through MAPK pathway as LIPUS enhanced extracellular signal-regulated kinase (ERK) 1/2 expression. Also, this effect is evidenced by the fact that methyl ethyl ketone (MEK) 1/2 inhibitor treatment suppressed the upregulation of COX-2 mRNA expression induced by LIPUS [8]. The integrin/Ras/MAPK pathway is a well-accepted general pathway that modulates cell proliferation.

LIPUS suppressed adipogenic differentiation of both adipogenic progenitor cell and mesenchymal stem cell (MSC) lines represented by impaired lipid droplet appearance and decreased gene expression of peroxisome proliferator-activated receptor γ2 (Pparg2) and fatty acid-binding protein 4 (Fabp4). Phosphorylation level of peroxisome proliferator-activated receptor γ2 protein was downregulated by LIPUS through the inhibition of its transcriptional activity. LIPUS also induced phosphorylation of cancer thyroid oncogene/tumor progression locus 2 (Cot/Tpl2) kinase, which was related to the phosphorylation of mitogen-activated kinase kinase 1 (MEK1) and p44/p42 extracellular signal-regulated kinases (ERKs). Notably, Cot/Tpl2-specific inhibitor affects stimulatory effects of LIPUS on both adipogenesis and osteogenesis. Furthermore, the inhibition of Rho-associated kinase suppressed stimulatory effects of LIPUS on MSC differentiation and Cot/Tpl2 phosphorylation. This report indicates LIPUS response to Rho-associated kinase-Cot/Tpl2-MEK-ERK signaling pathway in adipogenic progenitor cell and MSC cells [9].

LIPUS induced extracellular ATP release at 1min stimulation. LIPUS-induced extracellular ATP activates P2X7 receptor and increases extracellular matrix proteins (ECMPs) and bone formation but not the activation of alkaline phosphatase. [3]. ATP activates purinergic receptors such as P2 receptors including G protein-coupled receptors and ligand-gated channels. Particularly, the P2X7 receptor is a nonselective cation channel permeable to Na^+, K^+, and Ca^{2+}. ATP and $2'(3)$-O-(4-benzoylbenzoyl) ATP (BzATP) are agonists of P2X7 that induce the opening of P2X7 channels causing the elevation in intracellular calcium and depolarization of the plasma membrane [10]. Osteoblasts express functional P2X7 receptors both in situ and in vitro [11]. In vivo studies have shown that $P2X7^{-/-}$ mice have reduced osteogenesis in load-bearing bones, suggesting the role of P2X7 in the skeletal bone response to mechanical stress [12, 13]. gene silencing P2X7 (shP2X7) cells was not induced ECMPs by LIPUS. Furthermore, LIPUS increased the concentration of extracellular phosphate and calcium via P2X7 [3]. Thus, LIPUS-induced extracellular ATP may be degraded by ATP-hydrolyzing enzymes such as transglutaminase 2 (TG2), which contribute to the elevation of phosphate concentration. Indeed, ATPases have been shown to mediate mineralization without ALPase activity [14]; TG2 acts as ATPase in a calcium-dependent environment [15]. Taken together, LIPUS strongly responds to mineralized bone formation via extracellular ATP and the mechanoreceptor of P2X7.

LIPUS also responds to lipopolysaccharide (LPS)-TLR4 pathway in osteoblasts. LPS rapidly induced mRNA expression of several pro-inflammatory cytokines and chemokines including IL-1α, IL-6, RANKL, CCL2, CXCL1, and CXCL10 in both mouse osteoblast cell line and calvaria-derived osteoblasts. Simultaneous treatment by LIPUS significantly inhibited mRNA induction of IL-1α, IL-6, RANKL, CXCL1, and CXCL10 by LPS. LPS-induced phosphorylation of ERKs, p38 kinases, MEK1/2, MKK3/6, IKKs, TBK1, and Akt was decreased in LIPUS-treated osteoblasts. Furthermore, LIPUS inhibited the transcriptional activation of NF-κB responsive element and interferon-sensitive response element (ISRE) by LPS. In a transient transfection experiment, LIPUS significantly inhibited TLR4–MyD88 complex formation [5]. LIPUS reduced the gene expression of TLR4 induced by LPS [7]. Thus, LIPUS exerts anti-inflammatory effects on LPS-stimulated osteoblasts by inhibiting TLR4 signal transduction. Particularly, LIPUS acts angiotensin II receptor type I (AT1) on inhibition of IL-1α production induced by LPS through the inhibision of NF-κB activation. AT1 is a receptor of angiotensin II (Ang II). AT1-mediated signaling involves G protein dependent and independent pathways. AT1 belong to three G protein subfamilies: Gq, Gi, and G12 [16]. Mechanical stress activated AT1 receptor via an independent mechanism of Ang II. Mechanical stress activates extracellular signal-regulated kinases and increases phosphoinositide production *in vitro* but also induces cardiac hypertrophy *in vivo* without Ang II [17]. LIPUS increased the expression of AT1. Mechanical stimulation also reduced Ang II in ventricular cells of adult Sprague Dawley rats [18]. LIPUS reduced Ang II mRNA expression [7]. These results showed that AT1 may be stimulated by LIPUS and not in response to Ang II or LPS. AT1 antagonist losartan and siRNA silencing AT1 (siAT1) blocked all the stimulatory effects of LIPUS on IL-1α production. Furthermore, LIPUS also reduced the nuclear translocation of NF-κB by LPS-induced IL-1α and IL-1α-mediated NF-κB translocation induced by LPS, whereas AT1 inhibition with losartan or siRNA-mediated knockdown blocked this effect. PLCβ inhibitor U73122 also recovered NF-κB translocation. These results suggest that LIPUS inhibits LPS-induced IL-1α via AT1-PLCβ in osteoblasts. These reports exhibit are in part of the signaling pathway of LIPUS on the anti-inflammatory effects of IL-1α expression.

Taken together, LIPUS may respond to mechanotransduction through various receptors and the signaling pathway in osteoblasts which are mechanosensitive cells.

2.2 Effectiveness of LIPUS on Osteogenesis and Osteoclastgenesis

LIPUS promote osteogenesis through the upregulation of extracellular matrix protein and osteogenesis-related transcription factors such as RUNX2 and osterix in osteoblasts [2, 3] and enhance osteogenesis while inhibiting adipogenesis in cultured mouse bone marrow cells [9]. LIPUS also induced osteogenesis through the increases of BMP-7 in human fracture hematoma-derived progenitor cells [19]. LIPUS stimulation enhanced cell viability and proliferation. LIPUS also HSP90 was upregulated, leading to dense mineralization in the osteoblast cell culture after 10 days [20]. These findings indicate that LIPUS affects cell viability or proliferation and differentiation in various types of osteoblasts in vitro. Many clinical and in vivo studies reported that LIPUS is a mechanical stimulation that accelerates healing and regeneration of bone fractures; it also promotes osseointegration of dental implant and is therefore used in clinical settings [21–25].

In osteoclasts, osteoclastic markers such as tartrate-resistant acid phosphatase (TRAP) and cathepsin K mRNA expressions were decreased by 3 h incubation after LIPUS exposure. Both osteoclastic and osteoblastic marker mRNA expression did not change at 6 and 18 h of incubation after LIPUS exposure. TUNEL staining showed that the number of apoptotic osteoclasts was significantly elevated by treatment with LIPUS at 3 h of incubation. These results conclude that LIPUS directly functions to osteoclasts and that LIPUS directly causes apoptosis in osteoclasts shortly after exposure [26]. In 3 h incubation after LIPUS exposure, LIPUS induced an osteoclast differentiation factor of receptor activator of nuclear factor kappa B ligand (RANKL) in osteoblasts [27]. These findings suggest that LIPUS induces osteoclastogenesis at short incubation after stimulation in osteoclasts and osteoblasts in vitro [28]. Interestingly, both osteoclastic and osteoblastic marker mRNA expression did not change at 6 and 18 h of incubation after LIPUS exposure [26]. Thus, these findings indicate that the treatment of long-term LIPUS expose has an effectiveness on bone regeneration, whereas the treatment of short-term LIPUS exposure has an effectiveness on orthodontic tooth movement.

2.3 Effectiveness of LIPUS on Inflammation in Osteoblasts

Previous study reported the effect of LIPUS initiated after inflammation stage on the process of bone-tendon junction (BTJ) healing in a rabbit model in vivo. Thirty-six rabbits undergoing partial patellectomy were randomly divided into two groups: control and LIPUS. The period of initial inflammatory stage is 2 weeks. LIPUS treatment was initiated at postoperative week 2 and continued until the patella-patellar tendon complexes were harvested at postoperative weeks 4, 8, and 16. LIPUS treatment beginning at postoperative week 2 played an anti-inflammatory role in BTJ healing. The LIPUS group showed more advanced remodeling of the lamellar bone and marrow cavity than the control group, histologically. The area and length of the new bone in the LIPUS group were significantly greater than the control group at postoperative weeks 8 and 16. LIPUS beginning at postoperative week 2 could accelerate bone formation

during the bone-tendon junction healing process and significantly improved the healing quality of BTJ injury [29]. LIPUS also stimulates chondrocyte proliferation and matrix production in explants of human articular cartilage obtained from donors suffering from unicompartmental osteoarthritis of the knee, as well as in isolated human chondrocytes in vitro. Stimulation of [35S]-sulfate incorporation into proteoglycans by LIPUS was higher in degenerative than in collateral monolayers as assessed biochemically and higher in explants as assessed by autoradiography. LIPUS decreased the number of cell nests containing 1–3 chondrocytes in collateral and in degenerative explants. LIPUS increased the number of nests containing 4–6 chondrocytes in collateral and in degenerative explants. This suggests that LIPUS stimulates chondrocyte proliferation and matrix production in chondrocytes of human articular cartilage in vitro [30]. LIPUS also suppressed matrix metalloproteinase MMP-13 upregulated by osteoarthritis in chondrocyte in vitro in previous studies [31–33]. These results suggest that LIPUS affects the cartilage tissue repair in osteoarthritis and temporomandibular joint (TMJ) disease.

LIPUS reduced LPS (from *P. gingivalis* or *E. Coli*)-induced pro-inflammatory cytokines and chemokines such as IL-1α, IL-6 RANKL, CCL2, CXCL1, and CXCL10 in osteoblasts. LPS-induced IL-1α was inhibited by LIPUS via the suppression of NF-κB-AT1 pathway [7]. However, LPS-induced IL-6 and RANKL was not mediated AT1 by LIPUS. LIPUS also suppressed LPS-induced IL-6 and RANKL through the cyclooxygenase-2 (COX-2)-prostaglandin E_2 (PGE_2) inhibitions. In summary, LIPUS has anti-inflammatory effects on pro-inflammatory cytokine and chemokine production in osteoblasts. Thus, LIPUS has an effectiveness of inflammatory bone disease that is infected with *P gingivalis*, such as periodontitis.

LIPUS might provide a feasible tool for bone regeneration, orthodontic tooth movement, cartilage tissue repair for TMJ disease patients, and anti-inflammatory effect on the patients of periodontitis. Thus, LIPUS has an effectiveness in dentofacial region as a treatment tool of dental field.

2.4 Effectiveness of LIPUS on Tissue Regeneration in Dentofacial Region

Oral and maxillofacial diseases affect millions of people worldwide. Tooth decay, periodontal disease, dental pulp infection, and inflammatory root resorption can result in total or partial tooth loss and alveolar bone loss and can seriously compromise human health and quality of life. In addition, osteoarthritis of the TMJ (TMJ-OA) is characterized by erosion of articular cartilage, which becomes soft, frayed, and thinned, resulting in condylar resorption and deformity [34]. Their prevalence rates have ranged from 3% to 7% of the adult population [35], but once the breakdown in the joint starts, TMJ-OA can be crippling, leading to a variety of morphological and functional deformities [36]. As no treatment remedy of severe TMJ-OA has been developed yet, currently the TMJ disk and the mandibular condyle have been the focus of tissue engineering efforts.

Orofacial structures are very unique in their development and function. Orofacial bones are derived from both neural crest and paraxial mesoderm; however, the skeletal bones are derived from mesoderm. Furthermore, orofacial tissues have limited and variable capacity for regeneration. For example, cementum has a very slow and weak regenerative capacity [37], and dental pulp has a limited capacity for regeneration because of limited apical blood supply [38]. However, human postnatal dental pulp and periodontal ligament tissues include mesenchymal stem cells (MSCs) to multilineage differentiation in vitro and generate related dental tissues in vivo. In particular, dental pulp stem cells display multifactorial advantages, such as a high proliferation rate, high viability, and easy induction to distinct cell lineages [39]. Growing evidence supports expanding the use of dental tissue-derived stem cells in cell therapy and tissue engineering [40].

Odontogenesis is a complex process involving a series of epithelial-mesenchymal interactions and odontogenic molecular cascades, process as yet not understood [41]. A tissue engineering approach has been proposed for recovering lost teeth [42, 43]. Various biocompatible materials have been used to create scaffolds for tooth engineering such as hydroxyapatite ceramics, collagen sponge, chitosan gel, polyglycolic acid, polylactic acid, and β-tricalcium phosphate [44–47]. Complex tooth-like structures have been generated by seeding tooth bud cells onto a tricopolymer scaffold [44]. The combination of dental pulp stem cells with hydroxyapatite-tricalcium phosphate powder also forms a dentin-like structure in vivo [48, 49]. The successful identification and combination of tissue engineering, scaffold, progenitor cells, and physiologic signaling molecules have enabled to design and recreate the missing tissue in its near natural form, compared to the restorative and prosthodontic approaches. Some limitations to MSC-based therapy include scarceness of their numbers and extended time needed in the lab to differentiate these cells into chondrogenic and osteogenic lineages. Furthermore, issues involving the control to shape, size, and eruption of the tooth still remain to be solved. Tooth is, indeed, a complex biological organ, whose formation requires an intricate cascade of molecular signals and gene expression. In addition, detailed characterizations of extracellular matrix composition, tooth pulp tissue, collagen fiber destruction, and remodeling are needed in order to identify the instructive signals and gradients needed. Taking together, these strategies for tooth regeneration may eventually meet the challenge of generating bioengineered teeth of predetermined size and shape.

In the TMJ, since the fibrocartilage covering both mandibular condyle and articular eminence is avascular and the articular disc is composed of basically the same avascular tissue, intra-articular synovial fluid provides nourishment to these fibrocartilaginous cells which also have limited ability to self-repair [50–52]. In addition, like other synovial joints, mandibular condylar cartilage facilitates articulation with the TMJ disc and reduces point loads on the underlying bone [53], but it is of the fibrous type and is therefore structurally different from the generally applied hyaline articular cartilage, which can produce and release hyaluronic acid into the synovial fluid.

LIPUS therapy stimulates stem cell growth and differentiation [54–56]. LIPUS can be an effective tool to enhance tissue engineering of mandibular condyles for many reasons. Importantly, LIPUS is the preferred method of mechanical stimulation, also reported as "preferred bioreactor" as it enhances angiogenesis [57–59]. This is especially relevant because vasculature is required to integrate the engineered tissue with the native surrounding tissue [60]. Recent studies showed that LIPUS enhances cell expansion and differentiation in tissue culture [38, 54, 58].

Furthermore, many studies have demonstrated the potential of using embryonic stem (ES) cells for tooth regeneration, but many concerns also raised by the use of ES cells, such as possible tumorigenesis, ethical issues regarding the use of embryos, and allogeneic immune rejection, make this approach problematic. The use of iPS cells may overcome most of these issues, but this technology is still in its infancy and includes many unknown behaviors.

References

1. Ito A, Aoyama T, Yamaguchi S, Zhang X, Akiyama H, Kuroki H. Low-intensity pulsed ultrasound inhibits messenger RNA expression of matrix metalloproteinase-13 induced by interleukin-1β in chondrocytes in an intensity-dependent manner. Ultrasound Med Biol. 2012;38 (10):1726–33. https://doi.org/10.1016/j.ultrasmedbio. 2012.06.005.
2. Takayama T, et al. Low-intensity pulsed ultrasound stimulates osteogenic differentiation in ROS 17/2.8 cells. Life Sci. 2007;80(10):965–71.
3. Manaka S, et al. Low-intensity pulsed ultrasound-induced ATP increases bone formation via the P2X7 receptor in osteoblast-like MC3T3-E1 cells. FEBS Lett. 2015;589(3):310–8.
4. Yang RS, et al. Regulation by ultrasound treatment on the integrin expression and differentiation of osteoblasts. Bone. 2005;36(2):276–83.
5. Nakao J, et al. Low-intensity pulsed ultrasound (LIPUS) inhibits LPS-induced inflammatory responses of osteoblasts through TLR4-MyD88 dissociation. Bone. 2014;58:17–25.
6. Kokubu T, et al. Low intensity pulsed ultrasound exposure increases prostaglandin E2 production via the induction of cyclooxygenase-2 mRNA in mouse osteoblasts. Biochem Biophys Res Commun. 1999;256(2):284–7.
7. Nagao M, et al. LIPUS suppressed LPS-induced IL-1alpha through the inhibition of NF-kappaB nuclear translocation via AT1-PLCbeta pathway in MC3T3-E1. J Cell Physiol. 2017;232(12). https://doi.org/10.1002/jcp.25777
8. Iwabuchi Y, et al. Effects of low-intensity pulsed ultrasound on the expression of cyclooxygenase-2 in mandibular condylar chondrocytes. J Oral Facial Pain Headache. 2014;28(3):261–8.
9. Kusuyama J, et al. Low intensity pulsed ultrasound (LIPUS) influences the multilineage differentiation of mesenchymal stem and progenitor cell lines through ROCK-Cot/Tpl2-MEK-ERK signaling pathway. J Biol Chem. 2014;289(15):10330–44.
10. Pelegrin P, Surprenant A. Pannexin-1 mediates large pore formation and interleukin-1beta release by the ATP-gated P2X7 receptor. EMBO J. 2006;25 (21):5071–82.
11. Panupinthu N, et al. P2X7 nucleotide receptors mediate blebbing in osteoblasts through a pathway involving lysophosphatidic acid. J Biol Chem. 2007;282 (5):3403–12.
12. Li J, et al. The P2X7 nucleotide receptor mediates skeletal mechanotransduction. J Biol Chem. 2005;280(52):42952–9.
13. Ke HZ, et al. Deletion of the P2X7 nucleotide receptor reveals its regulatory roles in bone formation and resorption. Mol Endocrinol. 2003;17(7):1356–67.
14. Nakano Y, Addison WN, Kaartinen MT. ATP-mediated mineralization of MC3T3-E1 osteoblast cultures. Bone. 2007;41(4):549–61.
15. Lorand L, Graham RM. Transglutaminases: crosslinking enzymes with pleiotropic functions. Nat Rev Mol Cell Biol. 2003;4(2):140–56.
16. Hunyady L, Catt KJ. Pleiotropic AT1 receptor signaling pathways mediating physiological and pathogenic actions of angiotensin II. Mol Endocrinol. 2006;20 (5):953–70.
17. Zou Y, et al. Mechanical stress activates angiotensin II type 1 receptor without the involvement of angiotensin II. Nat Cell Biol. 2004;6(6):499–506.
18. De Mello WC. Mechanical stretch reduces the effect of angiotensin II on potassium current in cardiac ventricular cells of adult Sprague Dawley rats. On the role of AT1 receptors as mechanosensors. J Am Soc Hypertens. 2012;6(6):369–74.
19. Lee SY, et al. Low-intensity pulsed ultrasound enhances BMP-7-induced osteogenic differentiation

of human fracture hematoma-derived progenitor cells in vitro. J Orthop Trauma. 2013;27(1):29–33.

20. Miyasaka M, et al. Low-intensity pulsed ultrasound stimulation enhances heat-shock protein 90 and mineralized nodule formation in mouse calvaria-derived osteoblasts. Tissue Eng Part A. 2015;21 (23–24):2829–39.

21. Gebauer D, et al. Low-intensity pulsed ultrasound: effects on nonunions. Ultrasound Med Biol. 2005;31 (10):1391–402.

22. Harrison A, et al. Mode & mechanism of low intensity pulsed ultrasound (LIPUS) in fracture repair. Ultrasonics. 2016;70:45–52.

23. Nolte PA, et al. Low-intensity pulsed ultrasound in the treatment of nonunions. J Trauma. 2001;51 (4):693–702. discussion 702–3

24. Roussignol X, et al. Indications and results for the exogen ultrasound system in the management of non-union: a 59-case pilot study. Orthop Traumatol Surg Res. 2012;98(2):206–13.

25. Warden SJ, et al. Acceleration of fresh fracture repair using the sonic accelerated fracture healing system (SAFHS): a review. Calcif Tissue Int. 2000;66 (2):157–63.

26. Suzuki N, et al. Low-intensity pulsed ultrasound induces apoptosis in osteoclasts: fish scales are a suitable model for the analysis of bone metabolism by ultrasound. Comp Biochem Physiol A Mol Integr Physiol. 2016;195:26–31.

27. Bandow K, et al. Low-intensity pulsed ultrasound (LIPUS) induces RANKL, MCP-1, and MIP-1beta expression in osteoblasts through the angiotensin II type 1 receptor. J Cell Physiol. 2007;211(2):392–8.

28. El-Bialy T, et al. The effect of low intensity pulsed ultrasound in a 3D ex vivo orthodontic model. J Dent. 2011;39(10):693–9.

29. Lu H, et al. The effect of low-intensity pulsed ultrasound on bone-tendon junction healing: Initiating after inflammation stage. J Orthop Res. 2016;34 (10):1697–706.

30. Korstjens CM, et al. Low-intensity pulsed ultrasound affects human articular chondrocytes in vitro. Med Biol Eng Comput. 2008;46(12):1263–70.

31. Li X, et al. Effect of low-intensity pulsed ultrasound on MMP-13 and MAPKs signaling pathway in rabbit knee osteoarthritis. Cell Biochem Biophys. 2011;61 (2):427–34.

32. Xia P, et al. Low-intensity pulsed ultrasound affects chondrocyte extracellular matrix production via an integrin-mediated p38 MAPK signaling pathway. Ultrasound Med Biol. 2015;41(6):1690–700.

33. Ji JB, et al. Effect of low intensity pulsed ultrasound on expression of TIMP-2 in serum and expression of mmp-13 in articular cartilage of rabbits with knee osteoarthritis. Asian Pac J Trop Med. 2015;8 (12):1043–8.

34. Tanaka E, Detamore MS, Mercuri LG. Degenerative disorders of the temporomandibular joint: etiology,

diagnosis, and treatment. J Dent Res. 2008;87 (4):296–307.

35. Carlsson GE. Epidemiology and treatment need for temporomandibular disorders. J Orofac Pain. 1999;13 (4):232–7.

36. Zarb GA, Carlsson GE. Temporomandibular disorders: osteoarthritis. J Orofac Pain. 1999;13 (4):295–306.

37. D'Errico JA, et al. Immortalized cementoblasts and periodontal ligament cells in culture. Bone. 1999;25 (1):39–47.

38. Yoon JH, et al. Introducing pulsed low-intensity ultrasound to culturing human umbilical cord-derived mesenchymal stem cells. Biotechnol Lett. 2009;31 (3):329–35.

39. Kim BC, et al. Osteoblastic/cementoblastic and neural differentiation of dental stem cells and their applications to tissue engineering and regenerative medicine. Tissue Eng Part B Rev. 2012;18(3):235–44.

40. Lei M, et al. Mesenchymal stem cell characteristics of dental pulp and periodontal ligament stem cells after in vivo transplantation. Biomaterials. 2014;35 (24):6332–43.

41. Yang KC, et al. Fibrin glue mixed with platelet-rich fibrin as a scaffold seeded with dental bud cells for tooth regeneration. J Tissue Eng Regen Med. 2012;6 (10):777–85.

42. Henry PJ. Tooth loss and implant replacement. Aust Dent J. 2000;45(3):150–72.

43. Yelick PC, Vacanti JP. Bioengineered teeth from tooth bud cells. Dent Clin North Am. 2006;50(2):191–203. viii

44. Duailibi MT, et al. Bioengineered teeth from cultured rat tooth bud cells. J Dent Res. 2004;83(7):523–8.

45. Honda MJ, et al. Tooth-forming potential in embryonic and postnatal tooth bud cells. Med Mol Morphol. 2008;41(4):183–92.

46. Ohara T, et al. Evaluation of scaffold materials for tooth tissue engineering. J Biomed Mater Res A. 2010;94(3):800–5.

47. Sumita Y, et al. Performance of collagen sponge as a 3-D scaffold for tooth-tissue engineering. Biomaterials. 2006;27(17):3238–48.

48. Gronthos S, et al. Stem cell properties of human dental pulp stem cells. J Dent Res. 2002;81(8):531–5.

49. Gronthos S, et al. Postnatal human dental pulp stem cells (DPSCs) in vitro and in vivo. Proc Natl Acad Sci USA. 2000;97(25):13625–30.

50. Aoyama J, et al. Immunolocalization of vascular endothelial growth factor in rat condylar cartilage during postnatal development. Histochem Cell Biol. 2004;122 (1):35–40.

51. Fujisawa T, et al. A repetitive, steady mouth opening induced an osteoarthritis-like lesion in the rabbit temporomandibular joint. J Dent Res. 2003;82(9):731–5.

52. Tanaka E, et al. Vascular endothelial growth factor plays an important autocrine/paracrine role in the progression of osteoarthritis. Histochem Cell Biol. 2005;123(3):275–81.

53. Singh M, Detamore MS. Tensile properties of the mandibular condylar cartilage. J Biomech Eng. 2008;130(1):011009.

54. Angle SR, et al. Osteogenic differentiation of rat bone marrow stromal cells by various intensities of low-intensity pulsed ultrasound. Ultrasonics. 2011;51 (3):281–8.

55. Azuma Y, et al. Low-intensity pulsed ultrasound accelerates rat femoral fracture healing by acting on the various cellular reactions in the fracture callus. J Bone Miner Res. 2001;16(4):671–80.

56. El-Bialy T, et al. Ultrasound effect on neural differentiation of gingival stem/progenitor cells. Ann Biomed Eng. 2014;42(7):1406–12.

57. Al-Daghreer S, et al. Effect of low-intensity pulsed ultrasound on orthodontically induced root resorption in beagle dogs. Ultrasound Med Biol. 2014;40 (6):1187–96.

58. Nakamura T, et al. Low-intensity pulsed ultrasound reduces the inflammatory activity of synovitis. Ann Biomed Eng. 2011;39(12):2964–71.

59. Young SR, Dyson M. The effect of therapeutic ultrasound on angiogenesis. Ultrasound Med Biol. 1990;16 (3):261–9.

60. Romano CL, Romano D, Logoluso N. Low-intensity pulsed ultrasound for the treatment of bone delayed union or nonunion: a review. Ultrasound Med Biol. 2009;35(4):529–36.

Application of LIPUS for Bone Healing

3

Karima Mansjur and Eiji Tanaka

Abstract

Therapeutic low-intensity pulsed ultrasound (LIPUS) has been used to enhance bone healing caused by fracture in human and animal models, and it has been well accepted in accelerating tibial fracture healing, by delivering mechanical stimulation by means of LIPUS at an intensity of 30 mW/cm^2, with 200-ms pulses generated at a frequency of 1.5 MHz. For not only normal bone fracture but also for complex bone fractures in the presence of metabolic bone diseases such as diabetes mellitus (DM) and osteoporosis (OP), LIPUS might promote bone healing with increased mechanical strength and callus size together with reduced healing times. This implies that LIPUS can be a promising therapeutic tool for accelerating the fracture healing process. However, there has been still a controversy about the effects of LIPUS in human trials. Therefore, well-designed and precise clinical studies are needed to operate for further applications in tissue engineering.

K. Mansjur
Department of Orthodontics and Dentofacial Orthopedics, Institute of Biomedical Sciences, Tokushima University Graduate School, Tokushima, Japan

E. Tanaka (✉)
Department of Orthodontics and Dentofacial Orthopedics, Institute of Biomedical Sciences, Tokushima University Graduate School, Tokushima, Japan

Department of Orthodontics, King Abdulaziz University, Jeddah, Saudi Arabia
e-mail: etanaka@tokushima-u.ac.jp

3.1 Introduction

Therapeutic pulsed ultrasound has been used to enhance bone healing caused by fracture in humans and a variety of animal models [1]. In clinical treatment, it has been used in accelerating tibial fracture healing, by delivering mechanical stimulation by means of acoustic waves at an intensity of 30 mW/cm^2, with 200-ms pulses generated at a frequency of 1.5 MHz. The use of low-dose ultrasound was shown to stimulate bone healing with minimal heating effects. This was first reported by Maintz [2] after radius osteotomy in rabbits.

In 1952, Corradi and Cozzolino first stated that continuous wave of ultrasound could stimulate callus bone formation in a circular fracture rabbit model. In the next year, they proved in eight patients that the ultrasound wave was harmless and could generate an enhancement in their periosteal callus, and this became the first evidence of ultrasound application for fracture healing [3]. In 1983, Duarte first used low-intensity pulsed ultrasound (LIPUS) to stimulate bone healing in osteotomized rabbit fibulae [4]. Concurrently, Xavier and Duarte [5] effectively applied LIPUS to initiate healing of human fractures.

© Springer International Publishing AG, part of Springer Nature 2018
T. El-Bialy et al. (eds.), *Therapeutic Ultrasound in Dentistry*,
https://doi.org/10.1007/978-3-319-66323-4_3

Heckman and Kristiansen [6, 7] accomplished two laborious, double-blind, randomized, prospective, placebo-controlled clinical trials and discovered that the rate of healing of fresh fractures was accelerated by noninvasive exposure of LIPUS. The first trial examined the efficiency of ultrasound on closed or Grade-I open tibial shaft fractures, and the second trial tested the efficiency of ultrasound on dorsally angulated fractures. The patients on their trials had been exposed to ultrasound with an intensity of 30 mW/cm^2 for 20 min/day at home lasting for 10 weeks, as an auxiliary to conservative manipulation treatment with a cast. Effects of the treatment showed that the particular ultrasound could accelerate the healing of fractures and decrease the loss of reduction during fracture healing, and no serious complications were found associated with the use of ultrasound device. Afterward, the effect of LIPUS on bone healing was clinically established for fresh fractures in the 1990s together with non-union case and became approved by the Food and Drug Administration (FDA) for the treatment of fresh fractures in 1994 and for established non-unions in 2000 [6, 8, 9].

Busse et al. [10] performed a meta-analysis of six randomized controlled trials (RCTs): LIPUS was found to shorten the healing time by 64 days for fractures treated conservatively than that in the untreated control. Comparable positive effects were observed in tibial and distal radius fractures [11], complex tibial fractures [12], and scaphoid fractures [13]. In a review of the clinical evidence for fracture healing, Pounder and Harrison [14] reported that characteristically and widely used LIPUS at a frequency of 1.5 MHz with an intensity of 30 mW/cm^2 and a pulse rate of 20% could accelerate the healing time by up to 40% in fresh tibia, radius, and scaphoid fractures and that it was shown to be efficient to solve all types of non-unions of all ages. Urita et al. [15] showed that LIPUS shortens the cortical union time by 27% and endosteal union by 18% after forearm (radial or ulnar) bone shortening and osteotomies. Lately, Zura et al. [16] performed a cohort study of 4190 patients over 60 years old with fracture risk factors treated by LIPUS found to exhibit identical heal rates to the full population.

3.2 The Mode of Action of LIPUS in Fracture Repair

1. Effect of LIPUS in normal animal models of fracture repair
   For a better understanding of the effect of LIPUS on fracture repair, several preclinical animal models have been used to replicate the clinical setting. One such experimental in vivo model was made treating fractures at different time points of healing. Azuma et al. [17] created a rat closed femoral fracture in both hindlimbs with right femur exposed to LIPUS and left femur without LIPUS as control. Experimental animals were divided into four groups according to the timing and duration of the treatment. The authors considered this exposure schedule representing the hematoma, soft callus, and mineralization phases of fracture repair. Rats were treated with LIPUS for 20 min/day as follows: phase 1 group which received LIPUS for 20 min/day (from day 1 to 8 after fracture), phase 2 group which received LIPUS from day 9 to 18 after fracture, phase 3 group which received LIPUS from day 17 to 24 after fracture, and the last group which received LIPUS from days 1 to 24, throughout the fracture healing process. On day 25, animals were euthanized; radiographs and torsional biomechanical testing were performed to evaluate fracture healing. The maximal torque and stiffness in torsion of the fractured femur on the LIPUS-treated side were significantly greater than that of the left femur of control side in all groups ($p < 0.01$). This suggested that even short duration treatment with LIPUS during phase 1, 2, or 3 enhanced the mechanical properties of the fracture callus; nonetheless, treatment throughout the experimental period was most effective ($p < 0.05$). The histological results showed an acceleration of endochondral ossification and revealed that LIPUS-treated fracture sites at day 25 formed much more bone

than in the control at the same time point [17]. Freeman et al. [18] confirmed the acceleration of endochondral ossification by LIPUS exposure in in vivo study using a closed transverse mid-diaphyseal femoral fracture of rats. LIPUS was applied to the ipsilateral limb for 10 min/day, while the contralateral control limb received a sham exposure of LIPUS. The newly formed tissue was assessed by micro-CT each week for three weeks, with phasing thresholds which distinguished the un-mineralized tissue, less dense bone, calcified cartilage, and cortical bone. This method provided advanced substantiation of LIPUS influencing the fracture cascade, involving enhanced bone formation in the fracture gap and greater resorption of the "old" cortical bone. Histological observation also showed that in the LIPUS-treated fracture sites, the osteoclasts were significantly increased in number compared with controls, which indicates that LIPUS can influence the remodeling phase of fracture repair. The stimulation of osteoclastic action has been hypothesized as the consequence of increased concentrations of ATP released by LIPUS-treated osteoblasts into culture medium which was related to increased receptor activator of nuclear factor kappa B ligand (RANKL) and decreased osteoprotegerin expression [18].

2. Effect of LIPUS in Metabolic Bone Disease
   Fracture healing is a complex physiological process. The biological scheme consists of numerous specific sequential phases. These phases started with initial inflammatory phase with cell proliferation, continuing with the chondrogenic phase which involves the cartilage hypertrophy and angiogenesis and the osteogenic phase with replacement of cartilage into woven bone and subsequent remodeling. During the fracture healing process, numerous cells must participate and distribute sufficient and appropriate levels of inflammatory and bioactive molecules. Regardless of the complexity, most fractures heal naturally without any difficulties. However, numerous conditions are related with impaired bone

healing. These involve some extrinsic factors such as smoking, alcohol addiction, and prescribed medications like chronic steroid and chemotherapeutics. Smoking diminishes cell proliferation and angiogenesis, leading to reduced local availability of O_2 and antioxidant factors. Excessive alcohol consumption inhibits cell proliferation and osteoblast activity [19]. The presence of systemic disease such as diabetes mellitus (DM) and osteoporosis (OP) is also the associated factor with non-union and delayed union [7, 20].

LIPUS has been found to have a varied range of biological effects on tissues and has already been applied in the field of therapeutic medicine to enhance bone healing, resulting in increased mechanical strength and callus size together with reduced healing times even in the animal models of OP and DM [17, 21].

DM affects multiple phases in fracture healing, with its inherent morbidity of delayed bone healing and non-union. For example, DM Wistar rats and Long Evans rats with streptozotocin-induced (STZ) DM showed decreased cellular proliferation especially in the early phases of fracture healing. Furthermore, in the late phases of fracture healing, impaired mechanical strength and stiffness were observed [22, 23]. Gebauer et al. [24] investigated the healing effect of LIPUS on mid-diaphyseal femoral fractures in DM model rats. Although LIPUS had only diminutive effect on the early proliferative phase of fracture healing, its application did result in enhanced mechanical strength [24]. Furthermore, Coords et al. [25] evaluated the effects of daily application of LIPUS on mid-diaphyseal femoral fracture growth factor expression, cartilage formation, and neovascularization in DM Wistar rats. As the result, LIPUS was shown to increase growth factor expression, cartilage formation, and fracture callus neovascularization, indicating a potential role of LIPUS as an adjunct for DM fracture treatment [25].

Getting older, our bones are likely to lose volume and mineral density, resulting in decreasing bone strength. In older people, OP is a common condition that currently affects over 10 million people worldwide. OP occurs when bones lose mineral components more quickly or when replacement occurs too slowly, leading to weak and fragile bones. It has often developed unnoticed over many years without symptoms and discomfort until a bone fracture occurs. Due to excessive bone resorption and deficient bone formation, OP bone fractures have been associated with decreased callus quality, prolonged healing times, and non-unions in some cases [26–29]. Arai et al. [30] first reported clinical trial of LIPUS exposure to five OP bedridden patients. Daily exposure of LIPUS was applied for 4 weeks to the ipsilateral neck femur and resulted in approximate 8.9% increase in bone mineral density (BMD) compared with the baseline, while BMD on the contralateral non-treated side was reduced by about 4.0% within the same period. This finding indicates an anabolic effect of LIPUS in intact OP bone [30]. The first controlled study investigating the potential of LIPUS as a treatment of OP was conducted by Warden et al. [31]. This study examined the effect of LIPUS on hindlimb (distal femoral and proximal tibial) bone loss following ovariectomy (OVX) in rodents.

In the same year, Warden et al. [32] conducted the first controlled study of LIPUS effectiveness on OP patients. The aim of this study was to investigate whether LIPUS could prevent calcaneal OP in individuals succeeding spinal cord injury (SCI) to the extent observed by Arai et al. [30]. Fifteen patients with a 1–6-month history of SCI were enrolled. Active ultrasound signal with a 10 μsec burst of 1.0 MHz sine waves repeating at the frequency of 3.3 kHz with an intensity of 30 mW/cm^2 was introduced to one heel for 20 min/day, and the contralateral heel was treated with inactive LIPUS throughout 6 weeks. Bone status was assessed at the baseline and following the intervention period by dual-energy X-ray absorptiometry and quantitative ultrasound. There were no differences between active and inactive ultrasound-treated calcanei for any skeletal measure ($p > 0.05$). Opposed with the findings of Arai et al. [30], this finding demonstrated that LIPUS was unable to protect against SCI-induced calcaneal bone changes.

This may primarily relate to the inability of ultrasound to effectively penetrate the outer cortex of bone due to its acoustic properties and the intact OP bone might be less sensitive to LIPUS than isolated bone cells and defective bone. Being the first controlled study of the effect of ultrasound on OP patients, this finding did not completely exclude LIPUS as an intervention for osteoporosis [32].

On the contrary, Carvalho and Cliquet [33] performed a study to confirm the effects of LIPUS on OP bones. Rats were divided into two groups: non-treated and treated groups. In the treated group, rats were stimulated by LIPUS for 20 min/day for contiguous 20 days. The transducer included the femoral neck up to the distal third of the femur. More new bone formation and enhanced microarchitecture in treated group were observed than non-treated group [33]. Similar finding was reported by Wu et al. [34] who found that LIPUS had an anabolic effect on bone formation in an OP animal model. Using LIPUS at a frequency of 1.0 MHz with an intensity of 30 mW/cm^2 for 20 min/day, the right femur was treated with LIPUS (Sham-LIPUS and OVX-LIPUS) and the left femur was untreated (Sham-CON and OVX-CON). The wet weight of the femur increased in OVX rats with LIPUS stimulation. Morphological images showed an increase in trabecular spongiosa in the OVX-LIPUS group [34]. Woo et al. [35], using 14-week-old OVX imprinting control region (ICR) mice, also demonstrated that the elastic modulus in LIPUS-treated limbs was generally enhanced by an increased bone quality, compared to the control group. These studies suggested that LIPUS could prevent bone loss in OP and that LIPUS may be a promising treatment for OP.

The first animal study to depict the efficacy of LIPUS on OP fracture healing was performed by Cheung et al. [36]. Experiment was conducted on 120 female Sprague-Dawley (SD) rats that were divided into four groups—Sham OVX with LIPUS treatment (Sham-T), Sham OVX control (Sham-C), OVX with LIPUS treatment (OVX-T), and OVX control (OVX-C). Closed femoral midshaft fractures then were created, and LIPUS pulsed at a frequency of 1.5 MHz with an intensity of 30 mW/cm^2 was exposed 20 min/day and 5 days/week for durations of 2, 4, or 8 weeks, at which time radiography, BMD, microarchitecture measurement, histomorphometry, and mechanical testing were performed. Results indicated that two treated groups (Sham-T and OVX-T) showed significantly enhanced callus formation, faster mineralization, and better remodeling than the corresponding control groups (Sham-C and OVX-C) [36].

The effect of LIPUS on stimulation of bone healing in OP fracture and prevention of OP fracture has been extensively studied. Some fractures can heal on their own within 6–8 weeks without specific treatment to repair the fracture, depending on which bone is broken and how severe the OP condition. Nevertheless, there are cases in which bone union is not achieved even with the use of LIPUS, and it is challenging to judge the most suitable timing for repeated surgery. A large physical, mental, and social burden is placed on the patient when repeated surgery is needed.

The other patients with OP bone fractures get better with nonsurgical treatments such as limited use of anti-resorptive or anabolic medications; however, considerably longer time is required to fracture healing compared to healthy bone fracture. Furthermore, hospitalization for 6–8 weeks may make the patients bedridden. Therefore, treatments that can enhance callus formation and shorten the fracture healing time are indispensable for OP fracture patients without experiencing any treatment for OP.

Various anti-resorptive or anabolic drugs have been investigated for their capacity to inhibit excessive bone resorption or to accelerate new bone formation in OP bones. The latter includes estrogen, selective estrogen receptor modulators, calcitonin, bisphosphonates (BPs), and intermittently administered human parathyroid hormone (PTH) [37, 38]. In particular, PTH which plays multiple roles in calcium homeostasis and bone remodeling has been shown to increase bone remodeling by enhancing bone formation rather than bone resorption, thereby leading to an increase in bone mass, and improve bone microarchitecture [39, 40]. Therefore, PTH is

well recognized as a prevention drug for OP fracture in postmenopausal women [41, 42]. However, these drugs are developed and used to prevent, but not treat, OP fractures. Recently, we for the first time demonstrated that the combined therapy of PTH (1–34) and LIPUS leads to acceleration of fracture healing on OP fracture (Fig. 3.1) and enhancement of bone properties through improved bone volume, faster replacement of osseous tissues through histological observation, and enhanced microarchitectural parameters compared with the individual treatment (Fig. 3.2). This implies that the combined treatment of PTH and LIPUS might be beneficial in OP fracture healing. Meanwhile, the combined therapy of PTH and LIPUS has no additive effects on OP fracture healing although the beneficial PTH effect might not be impaired by the LIPUS exposure to OP fracture site. Our results also suggest the necessity of further studies to determine clinical efficacy, safety, and response duration [41].

Our unpublished data also suggested that therapeutic effect of PTH on OP fractures can be obtained with less frequent administration or a lower dose of PTH in combination with LIPUS exposure (Figs. 3.1 and 3.2). Female, 24-week-old SD rats with OVX were divided into three groups: control group without any treatment, PTH 1st group, and LIPUS 1st group ($n = 8$ in each). For all rats, a tibial fracture was created at the midshaft. After fracture, the PTH 1st group received PTH for the first 3 weeks and LIPUS treatment during the last 3 weeks. The LIPUS 1st group received LIPUS exposure for the first 3 weeks and PTH administration during the last 3 weeks. Results of the LIPUS 1st group showed significantly higher BMD and trabecular bone integrity than the other two groups at weeks 5–6. Radiographic evaluation of fracture healing score and mean callus area showed that LIPUS 1st and PTH 1st groups had better healing processes than the control. In addition, two treatment groups exhibited significantly higher bending moment. Since BMD has been used for the quantitative assessment of the mechanical properties in the healing bone, BMD is considered a principal key for reflecting the degree of mineralization in the callus. That is to say, LIPUS exposure may

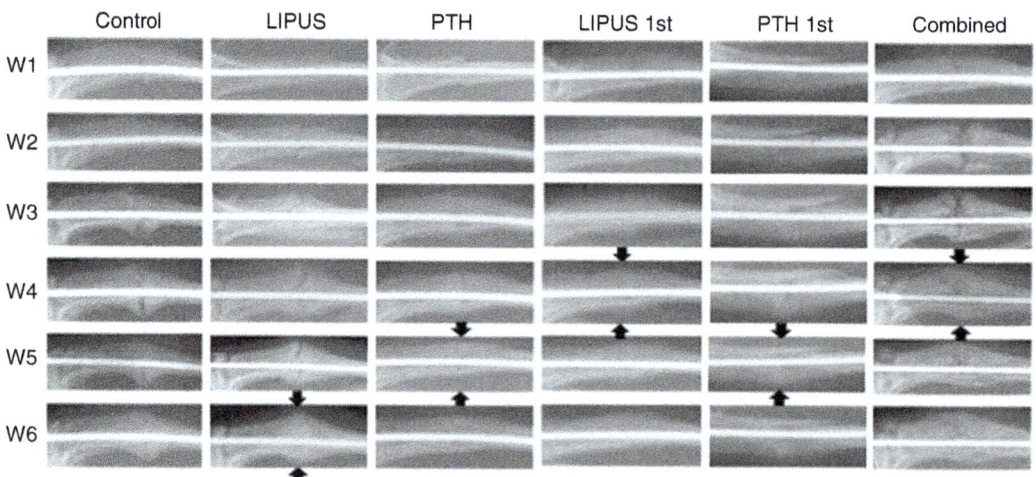

Fig. 3.1 Representative radiographic images of bilateral mid-diaphyseal tibial fractures in control, LIPUS, PTH, LIPUS 1st, PTH 1st, and combined groups at different time points. Note the increased radio-opacity of fractures in the combined and LIPUS 1st suggesting increased bone mineral density/callus depth. The fracture line on the original bone disappeared at week 4, in LIPUS 1st and combined groups, at week 5 in PTH and PTH 1st groups, and at week 6 in LIPUS groups. However, in control group, the fracture line still remained at week 6. Black arrows indicate fracture union. (Modified from Mansjur et al. [43])

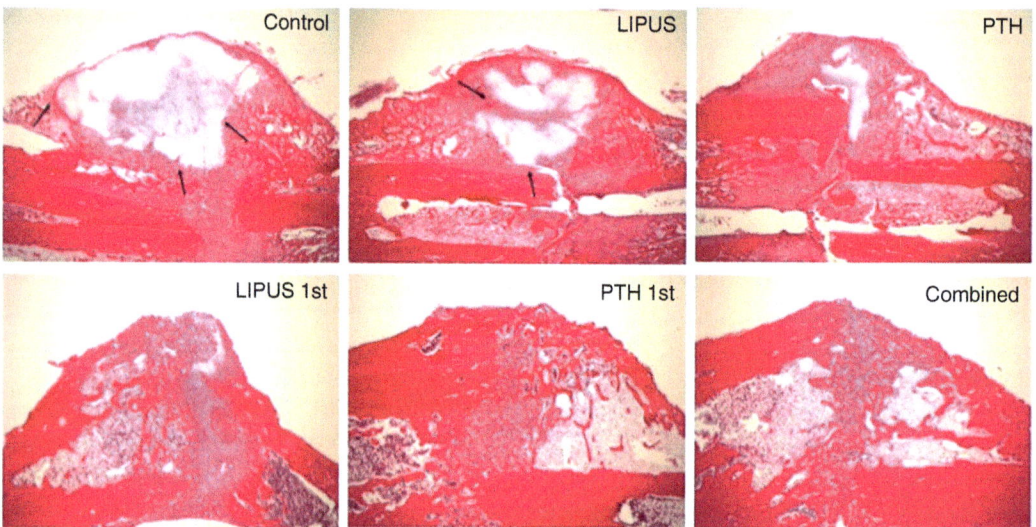

Fig. 3.2 Representative histological images of midshaft tibial fractures at 5 weeks post-fracture. Active endochondral ossification was continuing at week 5 in the control group, while the amount of chondroid tissues was reduced in treated groups (LIPUS, PTH, LIPUS 1st, PTH 1st, combined) and slightly replaced by osseous tissues (indicated by arrows). (Modified from Mansjur et al. [43])

stimulate earlier chondrogenesis, resulting in an earlier outcome of endochondral bone formation as well as advanced formation of bridging callus. This may result from the beneficial effects of the combination wherein LIPUS firstly accelerates callus formation and PTH induces replacement of fracture line by osseous tissues thereafter. Therefore, these findings might be confirmed by our hypothesis that the therapeutic effect of PTH on OP fractures can be obtained with less frequent administration or a lower dose.

In recent years, LIPUS has been paid attention as a noninvasive therapy that has little side effect. LIPUS has also been shown to enhance recombinant human BMP-2-induced bone formation at lower doses (1.2 and 6 μg) and callus maturation at 12-μg dose delivered on absorbable collagen sponge for bone repair in a rat critical-sized femoral segmental defect [44]. Therefore, LIPUS has much potential on clinical application since LIPUS can be used in combination with conventional pharmacotherapy.

3.3 Therapeutic Ultrasound and the Controversies

The current report provides much evidence that LIPUS has a positive effect on normal and delayed bone healing of animals such as rat models of OP and DM, implying that LIPUS can be a promising therapeutic tool for accelerating the fracture healing process. However, there has been still a controversy about the effects of LIPUS in human trials, such as fresh fractures, compressive fractures, and limb lengthening. Bashardoust Tajali et al. [45] performed a systematic review and meta-analysis to identify the clinical trials relevant to the effects of LIPUS on bone regeneration and retrieved seven human clinical trials on fresh fractures. They concluded that following LIPUS therapy, the time of the third cortical bridging of fresh fractures which correlated with increase in bone density was statistically earlier than control. Nonetheless, there was a dearth of satisfactory sufficient studies of LIPUS favorable effects on delayed unions and non-unions and no or weak differences evidence in acceleration of the fracture healing of LIPUS-treated and non-treated fractured bones [45–49]. The contentious reports of clinical success using LIPUS in repairing bone fractures could be due to the variations of the distance between the ultrasound transducer and the target organ and the depth of the target site in the target organ. In our previous study, when the distance

between the LIPUS transducer and the cells is less than 5 mm, attenuation of ultrasound intensity is negligible, and when the distance is more than 5 mm, attenuation is dependent on the distance and depth from the organ surface [50]. The variance in the proximity of the fracture bone ends to the LIPUS transducer could be one of the reasons for many contentious reports of clinical success using LIPUS in fracture healing. Note that most published papers with successful LIPUS therapy were operated on clinically reachable area of bones for LIPUS application. Furthermore, an attenuation rate of LIPUS waves absorbed by a specific tissue, depends to its density on the nature of the tissue. Bone commonly possesses the densest tissues in a given area, supporting the ultrasound waves to practically spotted areas where irregular bone may exist. Bones which are surrounded by thick muscle or in the case of deep bones showed less success by the treatment of LIPUS. As bone has the highest attenuation coefficients among biologic tissue types, when ultrasound waves are transmitted, it will hit an interface between two media with various acoustic blockades (i.e., soft tissue and bone), resulting in significant attenuation amount of waves might disappear during in transmission to living body due to the impedance mismatch. Three main separated issues that correlated with transmitted incident ultrasound waves are: impedance mismatch, attenuation, and the angle of incidence of waves [51–53]. Chung et al. [53] investigated the biological effects of four different incident angles performed in an vivo study using a rat femoral fracture model. LIPUS waves were transmitted in three different angles: 0°, 22°, 35°, and 48°, and the sham-treatment controls were compared. The results showed that callus mineralization, bridging and biomechanical properties were significantly enhanced in the 35° group over the control and 0° groups after week 8. LIPUS transmitted at 35°, which could be the critical application angle, showed the best enhancement effects among all the other groups. LIPUS transmitted at a critical application angle may enhance fracture healing significantly [53]. El-Bialy et al. [1] demonstrated in a research of rabbit mandibles that LIPUS power might be debilitated exponentially as the matter of length, and it concluded that there might be differences in clinical outcomes between studies regarding varieties in bone types and sizes.

3.4   Conclusions

The potential application of LIPUS for bone healing has been proved for many years. In the future, LIPUS may become an effective clinical procedure for the treatment of metabolic bone diseases such as osteoporosis and diabetes mellitus with the combination of anti-resorptive or anabolic medications. However, the controversies regarding LIPUS effects on fracture healing still remain to be investigated. Well-designed and precise clinical studies are needed for further applications in tissue engineering.

References

1. El-Bialy T, Royston T, Magin R, Evans CA, Zaki A-M, Frizzell LA. The effect of pulsed ultrasound on mandibular distraction. Ann Biomed Eng. 2002;30:1251–61.
2. Maintz G. Animal experiments in the study of the effect of ultrasonic waves on bone regeneration. Strahlentherapie. 1950;82:631–8.
3. Corradi C, Cozzolino A. Effect of ultrasonics on the development of osseous callus in fractures. Arch Ortop. 1953;66:77–98.
4. Duarte LR. The stimulation of bone growth by ultrasound. Arch Orthop Traum Surg. 1983;101:153–9.
5. Xavier CM, Duarte LR. Estimulacao ultra-sonica do calo osseo. Aplicacao Clinica Rev Bras Ortop. 1983;18:73–80.
6. Heckman JD, Ryabi J, McCabe J, Frey JJ, Kilcoyne RF. Acceleration of tibial fracture-healing by non-invasive, low-intensity pulsed ultrasound. J Bone Joint Surg Am. 1994;76:26–34.
7. Heckman JD, Sarasohn-Kahn J. The economics of treating tibia fractures. The cost of delayed unions. Bull Hosp Jt Dis. 1997;56:63–72.
8. Busse J, Kaur J, Mollon B, Bhandari M, Tornetta P 3rd, Schünemann HJ, Guyatt GH. Low intensity pulsed ultrasonography for fractures: systematic review of randomised controlled trials. BMJ. 2002;338:b351.
9. Kristiansen T, Ryabi J, McCabe J, Frey JJ, Roe LR. Accelerated healing of distal radial fractures with the use of specific, low-intensity ultrasound. A multicenter, prospective, randomized, double-blind, placebo-controlled study. J Bone Joint Surg Am. 1997;79:961–73.
10. Busse J, Bhandari M, Kulkarni A. The effect of low-intensity pulsed ultrasound therapy on time to fracture healing: a meta-analysis. Can Med Assoc J. 2002;166:437–41.
11. Cook S, Ryabi J, McCabe J, Frey JJ, Heckman JD, Kristiansen TK. Acceleration of tibia and distal radius fracture healing in patients who smoke. Clin Orthop Relat Res. 1997;337:198–207.
12. Leung K, Lee W, Tsui H, Liu PP, Cheung WH. Complex tibial fracture outcomes following treatment with low-intensity pulsed ultrasound. Ultrasound Med Biol. 2004;30:389–95.
13. Mayr E, Rudzki MM, Rudzki M, Borchardt B, Häusser H, Rüter A. Beschleunigt niedrig intensiver, gepulster Ultraschall die Heilung von Skaphoid-frakturen? Handchir Mikrochir Plast Chir. 2000;32:115–22.
14. Pounder NM, Harrison AJ. Low intensity pulsed ultrasound for fracture healing: a review of the clinical evidence and the associated biological mechanism of action. Ultrasonics. 2008;48:330–8.
15. Urita A, Iwasaki N, Kondo M, Nishio Y, Kamishima T, Minami A. Effect of low-intensity pulsed ultrasound on bone healing at osteotomy sites after forearm bone shortening. J Hand Surg. 2013;38:498–503.
16. Zura R, Mehta S, Della Rocca GJ, Jones J, Steen RG. A cohort study of 4,190 patients treated with low-intensity pulsed ultrasound (LIPUS): findings in the elderly versus all patients. BMC Musculoskelet Disord. 2015;16:45.
17. Azuma Y, Ito M, Harada Y, Takagi H, Ohta T, Jingushi S. Low-intensity pulsed ultrasound accelerates rat femoral fracture healing by acting on the various cellular reactions in the fracture callus. J Bone Miner Res. 2001;16:671–80.
18. Freeman T, Patel P, Parvizi J, Antoci V Jr, Shapiro IM. Micro-CT analysis with multiple thresholds allows detection of bone formation and resorption during ultrasound-treated fracture healing. J Orthop Res. 2009;27:673–9.
19. Tarantino U, Cerocchi I, Celi M, Scialdoni A, Cerrocchi I. Pharmacological agents and bone healing. Clin Cases Miner Bone Metab. 2009;6:144–8.
20. Oei L, Rivadeneira F, Zillikens M, Oei EH. Diabetes, diabetic complications, and fracture risk. Cur Osteoporos Rep. 2015;13:106–15.
21. Wang SJ, Lewallen DG, Bolander ME, Chao EY, Ilstrup DM, Greenleaf JF. Low intensity ultrasound treatment increases strength in a rat femoral fracture model. J Orthop Res. 1994;12:40–7.
22. Funk JR, Hale JE, Carmines D, Gooch HL, Hurwitz SR. Biomechanical evaluation of early fracture healing

in normal and diabetic rats. J Orthop Res. 2000;18:126–32.

23. Macey LR, Kana SM, Jinguishi S, Terek RM, Borretos J, Bolander ME. Defects of early fracture healing in experimental diabetes. J Bone Joint Surg. 1989;71:722–33.

24. Gebauer G, Lin S, Beam H, Vieira P, Parsons JR. Low-intensity pulsed ultrasound increases the fracture callus strength in diabetic BB Wistar rats but does not affect cellular proliferation. J Orthop Res. 2002;20:587–92.

25. Coords M, Breitbar E, Paglia D, Kappy N, Gandhi A, Cottrell J, et al. The effects of low-intensity pulsed ultrasound upon diabetic fracture healing. J Orthop Res. 2011;29:181–8.

26. Kubo T, Shiga T, Hashimoto J, Yoshioka M, Honjo H, Urabe M, et al. Osteoporosis influences the late period of fracture healing in a rat model prepared by ovariectomy and low calcium diet. J Steroid Biochem Mol Biol. 1999;68:3–8.

27. McCann R, Colleary G, Geddis C, Clarke SA, Jordan GR, Dickson GR, Marsh D. Effect of osteoporosis on bone mineral density and fracture repair in a rat femoral fracture model. J Orthop Res. 2008;26:384–93.

28. Namkung-Matthai H, Appleyard R, Jansen J, Hao Lin J, Maastricht S, Swain M, et al. Osteoporosis influences the early period of fracture healing in a rat osteoporotic model. Bone. 2001;28:80–6.

29. Hao YJ, Zhang G, Wang YS, Qin L, Hung WY, Leung K, Pei FX. Changes of microstructure and mineralized tissue in the middle and late phase of osteoporotic fracture healing in rats. Bone. 2007;41:631–8.

30. Arai T, Ohashi T, Daitoh Y, Inoue S. The effect of ultrasound stimulation on disuse osteoporosis. Trans Bioelectric Repair Growth Soc. 1993;13:17.

31. Warden SJ, Bennell KL, Forwood MR, McMeeken JM, Wark JD. Skeletal effects of low-intensity pulsed ultrasound on the ovariectomized rodent. Ultrasound Med Biol. 2001;27:989–98.

32. Warden SJ, Bennell KL, Matthews B, Brown DJ, McMeeken JM, Wark JD. Efficacy of low-intensity pulsed ultrasound in the prevention of osteoporosis following spinal cord injury. Bone. 2001;29:431–6.

33. Carvalho DCL, Cliquet A. The action of low-intensity pulsed ultrasound in bones of osteopenic rats. Artif Organs. 2004;28:114–8.

34. Wu S, Kawahara Y, Manabe T, Ogawa K, Matsumoto M, Sasaki A, Yuge L. Low-intensity pulsed ultrasound accelerates osteoblast differentiation and promotes bone formation in an osteoporosis rat model. Pathobiology. 2009;76:99–107.

35. Woo D, Ko C, Kim H, Seo JB, Lim D. Evaluation of the potential clinical application of low-intensity ultrasound stimulation for preventing osteoporotic bone fracture. Ann Biomed Eng. 2010;38:2438–46.

36. Cheung W, Chin W, Qin L, Leung KS. Low intensity pulsed ultrasound enhances fracture healing in both ovariectomy-induced osteoporotic and age-matched normal bones. J Orthop Res. 2012;30:129–36.

37. Cao Y, Mori S, Mashiba T, Westmore MS Ma L, Sato M, et al. Raloxifene, estrogen, and alendronate affect the processes of fracture repair differently in ovariectomized rats. J Bone Miner Res. 2002;17:2237–46.

38. Nozaka K, Miyakoshi N, Kasukawa Y, Maekawa S, Noguchi H, Shimada Y. Intermittent administration of human parathyroid hormone enhances bone formation and union at the site of cancellous bone osteotomy in normal and ovariectomized rats. Bone. 2008;42:90–7.

39. Kneissel M, Boyde A, Gasser JA. Bone tissue and its mineralization in aged estrogen- depleted rats after long-term intermittent treatment with parathyroid hormone (PTH) analog SDZ PTS 893 or human PTH (1–34). Bone. 2001;28:237–50.

40. Pettway GJ, Meganck JA, Koh AJ, Keller ET, Goldstein SA, McCauley LK. Parathyroid hormone mediates bone growth through the regulation of osteoblast proliferation and differentia- tion. Bone. 2008;42:806–18.

41. Black DM, Bilezikian JP, Greenspan SL, Wüster C, Muñoz-Torres M, Bone HG, Rosen CJ. Improved adherence with PTH(1–84) in an extension trial for 24 months results in enhanced BMD gains in the treatment of postmenopausal women with osteoporosis. Osteoporos Int. 2013;24:1503–11.

42. Henriksen K, Andersen JR, Riis BJ, Mehta N, Tavakkol R, Alexandersen P, et al. Evaluation of the efficacy, safety and pharmacokinetic profile of oral recombinant human parathyroid hormone [rhPTH (1–31)NH(2)] in postmenopausal women with osteoporosis. Bone. 2013;53:160–6.

43. Mansjur K, Kuroda S, Izawa T, Maeda Y, Sato M, Watanabe K, et al. The effectiveness of human parathyroid hormone and low-intensity pulsed ultrasound on the fracture healing in osteoporotic bones. Ann Biomed Eng. 2016;44(8):2480.

44. Angle SR, Sena K, Sumner DR, Virkus WW, Virdi AS. Combined use of low-intensity pulsed ultrasound and rhBMP-2 to enhance bone formation in a rat model of critical size defect. J Orthop Trauma. 2014;28:605–11.

45. Bashardoust Tajali S, Houghton P, MacDermid JC, Grewal R. Effects of low-intensity pulsed ultrasound therapy on fracture healing: a systematic review and meta-analysis. Am J Phys Med Rehabil. 2012;91:349–67.

46. Emami A, Petrén-Mallmin M, Larsson S. No effect of low-intensity ultrasound on healing time of intramedullary fixed tibial fractures. J Orthop Trauma. 1999;13:252–7.

47. Busse JW, Bhandari M, Einhorn TA, Schemitsch E, Heckman JD, Tornetta P 3rd, et al. Re-evaluation of low intensity pulsed ultrasound in treatment of tibial fractures (TRUST): randomized clinical trial. BMJ. 2016;355:i5351.

48. Handolin L, Kiljunen V, Arnala I. No long-term effects of ultrasound therapy on bioabsorbable screw-fixed lateral malleolar fracture. Scand J Surg. 2005;94:239–42.

49. Rue JP, Armstrong DW 3rd, Frassica FJ, Deafenbaugh M, Wickens JH. The effect of pulsed ultrasound in the treatment of tibial stress fractures. Orthopedics. 2004;27:1192–5.

50. Dalla-Bona D, Tanaka E, Oka H, Yamano E, Kawai N, Miyauchi M, et al. Effects of ultrasound on cementoblast metabolism in vitro. Ultrasound Med Biol. 2006;32:943–8.

51. Antich PP, Mehta S. Ultrasound critical-angle reflectometry (UCR): a new modality for functional elastometric imaging. Phys Med Biol. 1997;42:1763–77.

52. Mehta S, Antich PP. Measurement of shear-wave velocity by ultrasound critical angle reflectometry (UCR). Ultrasound Med Biol. 1997;23:1123–6.

53. Chung SL, Pounder NM, de Ana FJ, Qin L, Sui Leung K, Cheung WH. Fracture healing enhancement with low intensity pulsed ultrasound at a critical application angle. Ultrasound Med Biol. 2011;37:1120–33.

Application of LIPUS to Skeletal Muscles

4

Eiji Tanaka, Kumiko Nagata, and Nobuhiko Kawai

Abstract

Muscle injury affects muscle structure and function, resulting in muscle atrophy, contracture, and pain. The perfect repair of injured muscle tissue is later than the recovery of the movement and function of injured muscles, and the problems, such as re-injury, are subject to arise during the treatment of injured muscles. Low-intensity pulsed ultrasound (LIPUS) is reported to promote cell proliferation in fibroblasts and myoblasts. LIPUS might accelerate the inflammatory response immediately, bring early the phase of resolving inflammation in the injured muscle, recover the upregulation of myogenic transcription factors and skeletal muscle structural proteins, and accelerate skeletal muscle formation under inflammatory conditions. Taken together, LIPUS stimulation may be a better candidate as a medical remedy to promote myogenesis in inflammatory muscle states, such as muscle injury. Thus, LIPUS therapy may have considerable clinical potential for use in shortening the healing time of injured muscle. The next challenge in LIPUS therapy will be a treatment remedy for disease-related muscle atrophy in humans.

4.1 Introduction

Skeletal muscle is approximately 40–50% of human body weight, making this muscle the largest tissue mass and the most important protein reservoir in the body. Muscle mass maintenance is dependent on the balance between synthesis and breakdown of myofibrillar proteins [1].

Signal transduction pathways promote the synthesis and/or degradation of muscle proteins and mediate the regulation of muscle homeostasis as well as muscle hypertrophy or atrophy. Muscle atrophy, characterized by the progressive loss of muscle mass and strength, is a complex process that occurs as a consequence of various stress events, including neural inactivity, mechanical unloading, inflammation, metabolic stress, and elevated glucocorticoids [2]. The molecules and cellular pathways regulating skeletal muscle atrophy are still being discovered; however, multiple studies have shown that muscle atrophy in sepsis

E. Tanaka (✉)
Department of Orthodontics and Dentofacial Orthopedics, Institute of Biomedical Sciences, Tokushima University Graduate School, Tokushima, Japan

Department of Orthodontics, King Abdulaziz University, Jeddah, Saudi Arabia
e-mail: etanaka@tokushima-u.ac.jp

K. Nagata
Nagata Dental Clinic, Fukuoka, Japan

N. Kawai
Department of Orthodontics and Dentofacial Orthopedics, Institute of Biomedical Sciences, Tokushima University Graduate School, Tokushima, Japan

© Springer International Publishing AG, part of Springer Nature 2018
T. El-Bialy et al. (eds.), *Therapeutic Ultrasound in Dentistry*,
https://doi.org/10.1007/978-3-319-66323-4_4

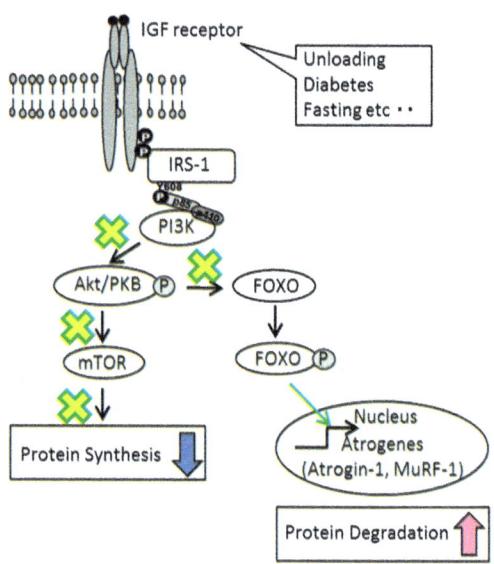

Fig. 4.1 Mechanism of muscle hypertrophy and atrophy

is primarily the result of increased protein breakdown [3, 4] via the ubiquitin-proteasome pathway [5, 6]. The IGF-1/PI3K/Akt signaling cascade plays an important role in the molecular mechanisms of muscle atrophy [7] (Fig. 4.1). The activity of the Akt pathway by unloading or chronic disease leads to low levels of phosphorylated FOXO in the cytoplasm. Both the phosphorylation and translocation of FOXO into nuclear are required for upregulation of atrogin-1/MAFbx and MuRF-1, which are ubiquitin ligases and critical mediators of atrophic myopathies [8]. Based on these findings, it is suggested that the inhibition of atrogin-1/MAFbx and MuRF-1 expression may prevent or reduce muscle atrophy.

Skeletal muscles contain a heterogeneous fiber type composition consisting of fibers with different physiological properties. These properties are mainly related to the expression of various myosin heavy chain (MHC) isoforms [9]. Sarcomeric myosin is a complex hexameric structure and is composed of four light chain (MLC) molecules,

named essential MLC and regulatory MLC and two MHC molecules (Fig. 4.2). The MLC molecules play a part in the conversion of chemical energy into movement. The MHC subunit contains the ATPase activity which provides energy to generate force for muscle contraction. There are several isoforms of the MHC molecules. These MHC isoforms, encoded by a multigene family, are in humans clustered at two distinct locations, two genes on chromosome 14 and 6 on chromosome 17 [10]. The MHC isoform genes found in humans include MHC-cardiac α, MHC-I, MHC-IIA, MHC-IIX, and MHC-IIB. Although MHC-cardiac α is normally expressed in the atrium of the heart, all the five types can be expressed in some mature jaw muscles [11].

The different isoforms of MHC are functionally unique and cannot be substituted for one another [12]. The main difference between the MHC isoforms is their rate of converting ATP into energy which determines the speed of actin–myosin detachment. There is a good correlation between the MHC isoforms and the contraction velocity of

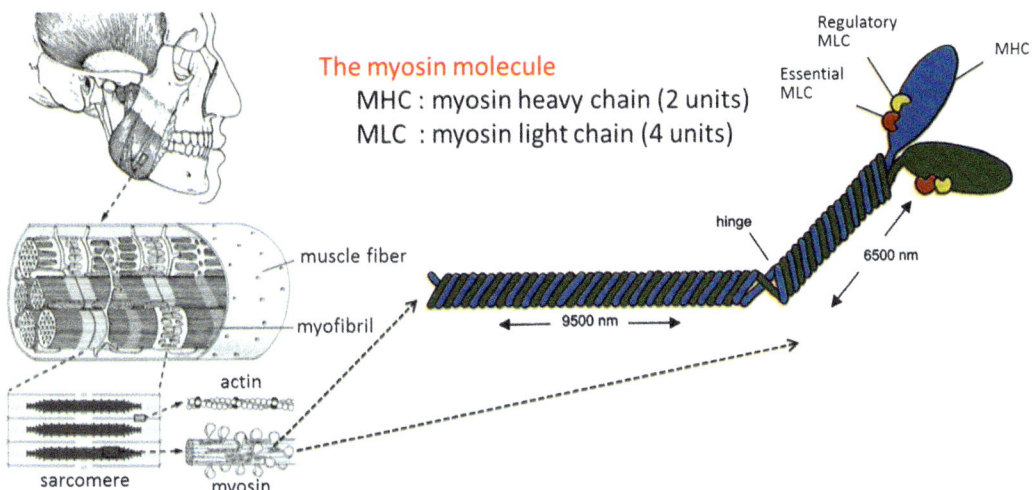

Fig. 4.2 The myosin molecule in skeletal muscles

fibers [13]. The contraction velocity increases successfully from fibers that contain predominantly MHC-I → MHC-IIA → MHC-IIX → MHC-IIB. The physiological property of muscle is related to the MHC phenotype. On this basis, muscle fibers are identified as infatigable-slow type I fiber and fatigable-fast type II fibers. For example, sprinter's muscle contains a lot of fast type II fibers, while marathon runner has few ones. Furthermore, muscle fibers are highly adaptive to environmental alterations, by changing one fiber type into another. For instance, during resistance training in humans the amount of MHC-IIX fibers decreased in favor of slower MHC isoforms, while disuse of the soleus muscle of the rat induced the conversion of MHC-I fibers into MHC-IIA fibers [14]. Similarly, the percentage of MHC-IIA fibers of the superficial masseter muscle in the soft-diet rats was significantly lower than that in the hard-diet rats and the opposite was true with regard to MHC-IIB fibers [15]. Furthermore, the cross-sectional area of MHC-IIX and -IIB fibers of the superficial masseter muscle was smaller in the soft-diet group than in the hard-diet group. This implies that the conversion of fiber types normally follows a strict order from MHC-I → MHC-IIA → MHC-IIX → MHC-IIB and vice versa [16].

Muscle strain, muscle pull, and muscle tear refer to damage to a muscle and/or its attaching tendons. In exercise, you can put undue pressure on muscles even during the course of normal daily activities. Muscle damage can be in the form of tearing of the muscle fibers and the tendons attached to the muscle. The tearing of the muscle can also damage small blood vessels, causing local bleeding, or bruising, and pain caused by irritation of the nerve endings in the area. Muscle injury is one of the muscle damages which occur most frequently in sports activities and daily life. Muscle injury affects muscle structure and function, resulting in muscle atrophy, contracture, and pain [17]. The perfect repair of injured muscle tissue is later than the recovery of the movement and function of injured muscles, and the problems, such as re-injury, are subject to arise during the treatment of injured muscles [18]. Therefore, the recovery of injured muscles needs the early repair of injured muscle tissue.

The recovery process of injured muscle can be divided into three distinct phases: the inflammation phase, the regeneration phase, and the remodeling phase. In the inflammation phase, small blood vessels, neutrophils, activated macrophages, and T-lymphocytes infiltrate the hematoma between the ruptured myofibers. Macrophages are involved in phagocytosis and removal of cellular debris and produce growth factors and cytokines [19, 20]. Cyclooxygenase-2 (COX-2) expression is increased by inflammatory stimuli, and COX-2 is typically considered pro-inflammatory. COX-2 pathways are involved in regulating pain, blood flow, platelet activation, leukocyte adhesion, and tissue infiltration. COX-2 induces prostaglandins that are involved in myoblast proliferation [21], differentiation [22], and fusion [23], in vitro. In vivo, the size of regenerating myofibers in freeze-injured tibialis anterior (TA) muscles of mice was decreased by COX-2-selective inhibitor starting before injury and was also decreased in COX-2 knockout (−/−) muscles [24].

The regenerative process of injured muscle is initiated by activating muscle satellite cells located in between muscle fiber and basal lamina [22]. In response to injury, satellite cells become activated, express paired-box transcription factor 7 (Pax7), and proliferate [23]. Pax7 is specifically expressed in nuclei of activating and proliferating satellite cells. The Pax7−/− mice develop limb muscles without satellite cells, and these mice are unable to grow or regenerate their limb muscles [24]. Thus, Pax7 is essential for the formation of satellite cells and muscle growth and regeneration. From the stage of satellite cells proliferating, satellite cells are called myoblasts. Myoblasts exit the cell cycle and undergo fusion to form myotubes. This process of myogenic differentiation is regulated by various myogenic regulation factors, such as MyoD and myogenin, which are the basic helix-loop-helix (bHLH) family of transcription factors and recognized as a biomarker, indicating the commitment of myoblastic cells to differentiation [25, 26].

It has been reported that low-intensity pulsed ultrasound (LIPUS) promoted cell proliferation in fibroblasts and myoblasts [27, 28]. Furthermore, LIPUS reduces inflammation and promotes regeneration in various injured soft tissues, such as collateral ligament injury [29] and injured skeletal muscle [27]. Thus, LIPUS therapy may have considerable clinical potential for use in shortening the healing time of injured muscle; however, the mechanism behind the effect of LIPUS on muscle healing has not been understood yet. It is hypothesized that LIPUS may provide mechanical stimulation to the cellular system associated with inflammatory substances and myogenic regulatory factors in injured muscle healing.

4.2 LIPUS Exposure to Injured Muscle

Nagata et al. [30] revealed that LIPUS exposure modulates inflammatory response and upregulates myogenic differentiation in inflammatory conditions in vitro and in vivo. For in vitro study, they cultured C2C12 cells in medium with or without TNF-α or IL-1β. After stimulation with cytokines, the cells received LIPUS or sham exposure. Furthermore, for in vivo study, the tibialis anterior (TA) muscle in C57BL/6 mice injured by cardiotoxin (CTX) was dissected after a series of LIPUS treatments and examined. LIPUS exposure system modified from a clinical device (BR Sonic-pro, ITO Co., Tokyo, Japan) was used both in vitro and in vivo. In vitro, this system consisted of a 9.6 cm^2 circular surface transducer and a culture flask. A pulsed ultrasound signal was transmitted at a frequency of 3 MHz with a spatially averaged intensity of 30 mW/cm^2 and pulsed 1:4 (2 ms on and 8 ms off). In vivo, the ultrasound exposure system was equipped with a circular transducer of 18 mm in diameter. A pulsed ultrasound signal was transmitted at a frequency of 1 MHz with a spatially averaged intensity of 150 mW/cm^2 and pulsed 1:4. Exposure of C2C12 cells to LIPUS resulted in downregulation of COX-2 mRNA and protein expression induced by TNF-α or IL-1β, and upregulated myogenin mRNA and protein depressed by TNF-α or IL-1β. In injured TA muscle induced by CTX, LIPUS caused increase of COX-2 mRNA at 1 day after LIPUS treatment but, at day 5, reduction of COX-2 mRNA and protein. At day 5, LIPUS caused increase of myogenin mRNA and protein, increase of fast myosin protein, and increase of Pax7-positive cells (Figs. 4.3a, b, c). At day 7, the cross-sectional area of myofibers in the LIPUS exposure side was significantly larger than that on the control side (Fig. 4.3d).

In their study, COX-2 gene expression was increased by LIPUS exposure at the early stage in the injured TA muscle by CTX; however, LIPUS decreased COX-2 gene and protein expression at the late stage in the injured TA

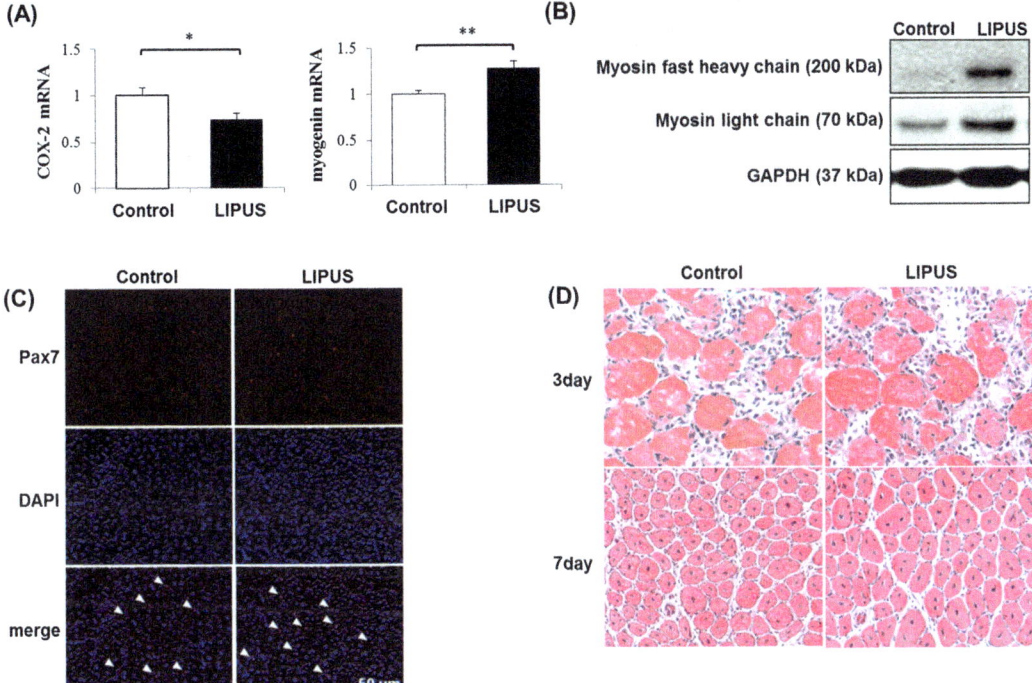

Fig. 4.3 LIPUS exposure to injured tibialis anterior muscle induced by cardiotoxin. (**a**) The expression of COX-2 and myogenin mRNA at 5 days after LIPUS exposure in the injured TA muscle. The expression of COX-2 and myogenin mRNA in the LIPUS-treated side was decreased compared to the control side. (**b**) Myosin fast heavy and light chain protein syntheses at 5 days after LIPUS exposure in injured muscle. The expression of fast heavy and light myosin chain protein in LIPUS-treated side was increased compared with that in the control side.

(**c**) Immunofluorescence for detecting Pax7 in the injured muscle at day 5. The number of Pax7-positive cells in the LIPUS side was markedly larger than that in the control side. (**d**) Microphotographs of the injured muscle by cardiotoxin at 3 and 7 days after LIPUS treatment. At 7 days after LIPUS exposure, the cross-sectional area of myofiber-centered nuclei in the LIPUS side increased significantly compared with that in the control side. (Modified from Nagata et al. [30])

muscle. Furthermore, the number of inflammatory infiltration cells in the LIPUS-treated side was decreased significantly compared with that in the control side at 5 days after LIPUS treatment. In C2C12 cells, although COX-2 expression increased significantly by TNF-α or IL-1β stimulus was not decreased at 1 h after LIPUS exposure, it was decreased to the control level at 3 h. These suggest that LIPUS exposure modulates inflammation in the injured muscle. The recovery process of the injured muscle begins from the inflammatory response first. Inflammation is an important phase of skeletal muscle healing. Muscle regeneration depends on various cellular events caused by a number of growth factors and cytokines [31].

However, persistence of inflammation often prevents the damaged muscle from regenerating efficiently. The inflammatory response must be resolved to allow muscle repair. In skeletal muscle, chronic administration of TNF-α or IL-1β induced weight loss and skeletal muscle wasting in rats [32]. In contrast, in injured rat skeletal muscle, LIPUS exposure reduced COX-2 expression and the number of leukocytes [33, 34]. Mechanical stimuli, such as cyclic tensile stress, also inhibited the expression of several pro-inflammatory genes controlled by NF-kB transcriptional activity, such as NOS2, COX-2, MMP1, and IL-1β in C2C12 cells or chondrocytes [35, 36]. Therefore, the biomechanical signals of LIPUS might not reduce the inflammatory response but bring early the phase of resolving inflammation.

In vitro studies demonstrated that TNF-α leads to the reduction of MyoD, myogenin, and MHC protein synthesis, resulting in the eventual inhibition of myotube formation [37, 38]. On the other hand, Chandran et al. [39] showed that cyclic tensile stress acts as a potent inhibitor of the intracellular actions by pro-inflammatory cytokines like TNF-α and upregulates myogenic transcription factors and skeletal muscle structural proteins despite the presence of strong pro-inflammatory conditions in C2C12 cells. It has been shown that mechanical stress such as stretch and cyclic tensile stress induced upregulation of myogenic regulatory factors in whole muscle model and culture model [40, 41] and that cyclic stretching promoted hypertrophy in cultured skeletal myotubes primarily through activating the PI3K/Akt/TOR pathway [42]. However, Nagata et al. [30] revealed that LIPUS could not accelerate the expression of the myogenic regulatory factor and induce hypertrophy in cultured skeletal myotubes in the absence of inflammation.

Therefore, it is concluded that LIPUS might accelerate the inflammatory response immediately, bring early the phase of resolving inflammation in the injured muscle, recover the upregulation of myogenic transcription factors and skeletal muscle structural proteins, and accelerate skeletal muscle formation under inflammatory conditions. Taken together, LIPUS stimulation may be a better candidate as a medical remedy to promote myogenesis in inflammatory muscle states, such as muscle injury.

4.3   Looking to the Future: Muscle Atrophy

Numerous diseases associated with chronic inflammation often result in skeletal muscle weakness and fatigue. Disease-related muscle atrophy and fatigue is an important clinical problem because acquired muscle weakness can increase the duration of hospitalization, resulting in exercise limitation. Furthermore, hospitalization for longer than 2 months may make the patients bedridden due to muscle disuse. Importantly, atrophy of masticatory muscles is also associated with decreased amount of a meal, resulting in a poor quality of life. Muscle atrophy is caused by an imbalance in contractile protein synthesis and degradation which can be triggered by various conditions including Type 2 Diabetes Mellitus (T2DM). Reduced muscle quality in patients with T2DM adversely affects muscle function and the capacity to perform activities of daily living and may increase the risk of premature mortality. Systemic inflammation initiated by obesity not only contributes to insulin resistance typical of T2DM but also promotes muscle atrophy via decreased muscle protein synthesis and increased muscle protein degradation. Therefore, if we can reduce inflammation in skeletal muscles, progress in muscle atrophy in T2DM patients might be restricted.

Despite its short history and the relatively few published reports, significant advances have already been made in muscle regeneration by LIPUS. While muscle regeneration may revolutionize the future of muscle atrophy and dystrophy, it will be absolutely necessary to remember the lessons of the past gleaned from decades of successes and failures with muscle regeneration. The next challenge in LIPUS therapy will be a treatment remedy for disease-related muscle atrophy in humans.

References

1. Attaix D, Baracos VE, Pichard C. Muscle wasting: a crosstalk between protein synthesis and breakdown signaling. Curr Opin Clin Nutr Metab Care. 2012;15:209–10.
2. Schiaffino S, Dyar KA, Ciciliot S, Blaauw B, Sandri M. Mechanisms regulating skeletal muscle growth and atrophy. FEBS J. 2013;280:4294–314.
3. Hasselgren PO, Talamini M, James JH, Fischer JE. Protein metabolism in different types of skeletal muscle during early and late sepsis in rats. Arch Surg. 1986;121:918–23.
4. Hasselgren PO, James JH, Benson DW, Hall-Angeras M, Angeras U, Hiyama DT, et al. Total and myofibrillar protein breakdown in different types of rat skeletal muscle: effects of sepsis and regulation by insulin. Metabolism. 1989;38:634–40.

5. Tiao G, Fagan JM, Samuels N, James JH, Hudson K, Lieberman M, et al. Sepsis stimulates nonlysosomal, energy-dependent proteolysis and increases ubiquitin mRNA levels in rat skeletal muscle. J Clin Invest. 1994;94:2255–64.

6. Tiao G, Hobler S, Wang JJ, Meyer TA, Luchette FA, Fischer JE, Hasselgren PO. Sepsis is associated with increased mRNAs of the ubiquitin-proteasome proteolytic pathway in human skeletal muscle. J Clin Invest. 1997;99:163–8.

7. Sandri M, Sandri C, Gilbert A, Skurk C, Calabria E, Picard A, et al. Foxo transcription factors induce the atrophy-related ubiquitin ligase atrogin-1 and cause skeletal muscle atrophy. Cell. 2004;117:399–412.

8. Stitt TN, Drujan D, Clarke BA, Panaro F, Timofeyva Y, Kline WO, et al. The IGF-1/PI3K/Akt pathway prevents expression of muscle atrophy-induced ubiquitin ligases by inhibiting FOXO transcription factors. Mol Cell. 2004;14:395–403.

9. Cobos AR, Segade LA, Fuentes I. Muscle fiber types in the suprahyoid muscles of the rat. J Anat. 2001;198:283–94.

10. Weiss A, Schiaffino S, Leinwand LA. Comparative sequence analysis of the complete human sarcomeric myosin heavy chain family: implications for functional diversity. J Mol Biol. 1999;290:61–75.

11. Monemi M, Eriksson PO, Dubail I, Bulter-Browne GS, Thornell LE. Fetal myosin heavy chain increases in the human masseter muscle during aging. FEBS Lett. 1996;386:87–90.

12. Allen DL, Harrison BC, Leinwand LA. Inactivation of myosin heavy chain genes in the mouse: diverse and unexpected phenotypes. Microsc Res Tech. 2000;50:492–9.

13. Bottinelli R, Canepari M, Pellegrino MA, Reggiani C. Force-velocity properties of human skeletal muscle fibres: myosin heavy chain isoform and temperature dependence. J Physiol. 1996;495:573–86.

14. Oishi Y, Ishihara A, Yamamoto H, Miyamoto E. Hindlimb suspension induces the expression of multiple myosin heavy chain isoforms in single fibres of the rat soleus muscle. Acta Physiol Scand. 1998;162:127–34.

15. Kawai N, Sano R, Korfage JAM, Nakamura S, Kinouchi N, Kawakami E, et al. Adaptation of rat jaw muscle fibers in postnatal development with a different food consistency: an immnohistochemical and EMG study. J Anat. 2010;216:717–23.

16. Schiaffino S, Reggiani C. Myosin isoforms in mammalian skeletal muscle. J Appl Physiol. 1994;77:493–501.

17. Madhavan S, Shields RK. Weight-bearing exercise accuracy influences muscle activation strategies of the knee. J Neurol Phys Ther. 2007;31:12–9.

18. Iwata A, Fuchioka S, Hiraoka K, Masuhara M, Kami K. Characteristics of locomotion, muscle strength, and muscle tissue in regenerating rat skeletal muscles. Muscle Nerve. 2010;41:694–701.

19. Gebauer D, Correll J. Pulsed low-intensity ultrasound: a new salvage procedure for delayed unions and nonunions after leg lengthening in 23 children. J Pediatr Orthop. 2005;6:750–4.

20. Robertson TA, Maley MA, Grounds MD, Papadimitriou JM. The role of macrophage in skeletal muscle regeneration with particular reference of chemotaxis. Exp Cell Res. 1993;207:321–31.

21. Zalin RJ. The role of hormones and prostanoids in the in vitro proliferation and differentiation of human myoblasts. Exp Cell Res. 1987;172:265–81.

22. Schutzle UB, Wakelam MJ, Pette D. Prostaglandins and cyclic AMP stimulate creatine kinase synthesis but not fusion in cultured embryonic chick muscle cells. Biochem Biophys Acta. 1984;805:204–10.

23. Eutwistle A, Curtis DH, Zalin RJ. Myoblast fusion is regulated by a prostanoid of the one series independently of a rise in cyclic AMP. J Cell Biol. 1986;103:857–66.

24. Bondesen BA, Mills ST, Kegley KM, Pavlath GK. The COX-2 pathway is essential during early stage of skeletal muscle regeneration. Am J Physiol Cell Physiol. 2004;287:475–83.

25. Naidu PS, Ludolph DC, To RQ, Hinterberger TJ, Konieczny SF. Myogenin and MEF2 function synergistically to activate the MRF4 promoter during myogenesis. Mol Cell Biol. 1995;15:2707–18.

26. Rawls A, Valdez MR, Zhang W, Richardson J, Klein WH, Olson EN. Overlapping functions of the myogenic bHLH genes MRF4 and MyoD revealed in double mutant mice. Development. 1998;125:2349–58.

27. Chan YS, Hsu KY, Kuo CH, Lee SD, Chen SC, Chen WJ, et al. Using low-intensity pulsed ultrasound to improve muscle healing after laceration injury: an in vitro and in vivo study. Ultrasound Med Biol. 2010;36:743–51.

28. Zhou S, Schmelz A, Seufferlein T, Li Y, Zhao J, Bachem MG. Molecular mechanisms of low intensity pulsed ultrasound in human skin fibroblasts. J Biol Chem. 2004;279:54463–9.

29. Takakura Y, Matsui N, Yoshiya S, Fujioka H, Muratsu H, Tsunoda M, et al. Low-intensity pulsed ultrasound enhances early healing of medial collateral ligament injuries in rats. J Ultrasound Med. 2002;21:283–8.

30. Nagata K, Nakamura T, Fujiwara S, Tanaka E. Ultrasound modulates the inflammatory response and promotes muscle regeneration in injured muscles. Ann Biomed Eng. 2013;41:1095–105.

31. St. Pierre BA, Tidball JG. Differential response of macrophage subpopulations to soleus muscle reloading after rat hindlimb suspension. J Appl Physiol. 1994;77:290–7.

32. Fong Y, Moldawer LL, Marano M, Wei H, Barber A, Manogue K, et al. Cachectin/TNF or IL-1 alpha induces cachexia with redistribution of body proteins. Am J Physiol. 1989;256:659–65.

33. Renno AC, Toma RL, Feitosa SM, Fernandes K, Bossini PS, de Oliveira P, et al. Comparative effects of low-intensity pulsed ultrasound and low-level laser therapy on injured skeletal muscle. Photomed Laser Surg. 2011;29:5–10.

34. Signori LU, da Costa ST, Neto AF, Pizzolotto RM, Beck C, Sbruzzi G, et al. Haematological effect of pulsed ultrasound in acute muscular inflammation in rats. Physiotherapy. 2011;97:163–9.

35. Markert CD, Merrick MA, Kirby TE, Devor ST. Nonthermal ultrasound and exercise in skeletal muscle regeneration. Arch Phys Med Rehabil. 2005;86:1304–10.

36. Agarwal S, Deschner J, Long P, Verma A, Hofman C, Evans CH, et al. Role of NF-kappaB transcription factors in antiinflammatory and proinflammatory actions of mechanical signals. Arthritis Rheum. 2004;50:3541–8.

37. Acharyya S, Ladner KJ, Nelsen LL, Damrauer J, Reiser PJ, Swoap S, et al. Cancer cachexia is regulated by selective targeting of skeletal muscle gene products. J Clin Invest. 2004;114:370–8.

38. Guttridge DC. Signaling pathways weigh in on decisions to make or break skeletal muscle. Curr Opin Clin Nutr Metab Care. 2004;7:443–50.

39. Chandran R, Knobloch TJ, Anghelina M, Agarwal S. Biomechanical signals upregulate myogenic gene induction in the presence or absence of inflammation. Am J Physiol Cell Physiol. 2007;293:267–76.

40. Lowe DA, Always SE. Stretch-induced myogenin, MyoD, and MRF4 expression and acute hypertrophy in quail slow-tonic muscle are not dependent upon satellite cell proliferation. Cell Tissue Res. 1999;296:531–9.

41. Rauch C, Loughna PT. Cyclosporin-A inhibits stretch-induced changes in myosin heavy chain expression in C2C12 skeletal muscle cells. Cell Biochem Funct. 2006;24:55–61.

42. Sakai N, Agata N, Inoue-Miyazu M, Kawakami K, Kobayashi K, Sokabe M, et al. Involvement of PI3K/Akt/TOR pathway in stretch-induced hypertrophy of myotube. Muscle Nerve. 2010;41:100–6.

Application of LIPUS to Periodontal Tissue Regeneration

Eiji Tanaka, Toshihiro Inubushi, and Tarek El-Bialy

Abstract

Exposure to ultrasound during the inflammatory phase of periodontal tissue repair leads to an acceleration of this phase, which may eventually lead to an anti-inflammatory effect by low-intensity pulsed ultrasound (LIPUS) exposure. LIPUS has also been shown to enhance collagen synthesis by fibroblasts. As a consequence, LIPUS may be a promising candidate of treatment remedy for periodontal diseases such as periodontitis and orthodontically induced root resorption. Recent in vitro studies suggested that LIPUS promotes osteogenic differentiation of human periodontal ligament (PDL) cells, which is associated with upregulation of Runx2 and integrin $\beta 1$ and activation of bone morphogenetic protein-smad signaling. Furthermore, recent in vivo studies have shown that LIPUS can enhance periodontal tissue repair and regeneration, especially if combined with the other treatment remedies for periodontal diseases such as guided tissue regeneration (GTR). These suggest that LIPUS could potentially enhance periodontal tissue repair and regeneration combined with GTR and provide therapeutic benefits in periodontal tissue regeneration.

5.1 Introduction

Periodontal ligament (PDL), located between the root surface (cementum) and alveolar bone, is composed of cells and extracellular compartment comprising collagenous and noncollagenous matrix components (Fig. 5.1). PDL consists of different cell populations, including fibroblasts, osteoblasts, cementoblasts, and undifferentiated mesenchymal cells, according to the location in PDL. For example, PDL includes precursor cells of cementoblasts at the perivascular area in the middle portion and shows greater differentiation toward the surface of the root [1]. Therefore, it has been generally accepted that PDL plays a central role in the maintenance of periodontal tissues by serving as a source of renewable progenitor cells.

One of the functions of PDL is to withstand and respond to mechanical stress induced by functional mandibular movements such as

E. Tanaka (✉)
Department of Orthodontics and Dentofacial Orthopedics, Institute of Biomedical Sciences, Tokushima University Graduate School, Tokushima, Japan

Department of Orthodontics, King Abdulaziz University, Jeddah, Saudi Arabia
e-mail: etanaka@tokushima-u.ac.jp

T. Inubushi
Genetic Disease Program, Sanford Children's Health Research Center, Sanford-Burnham Medical Research Institute, La Jolla, CA, USA

T. El-Bialy
Dentistry/Orthodontics and Biomedical Engineering, University of Alberta, Edmonton, Alberta, Canada

© Springer International Publishing AG, part of Springer Nature 2018
T. El-Bialy et al. (eds.), *Therapeutic Ultrasound in Dentistry*,
https://doi.org/10.1007/978-3-319-66323-4_5

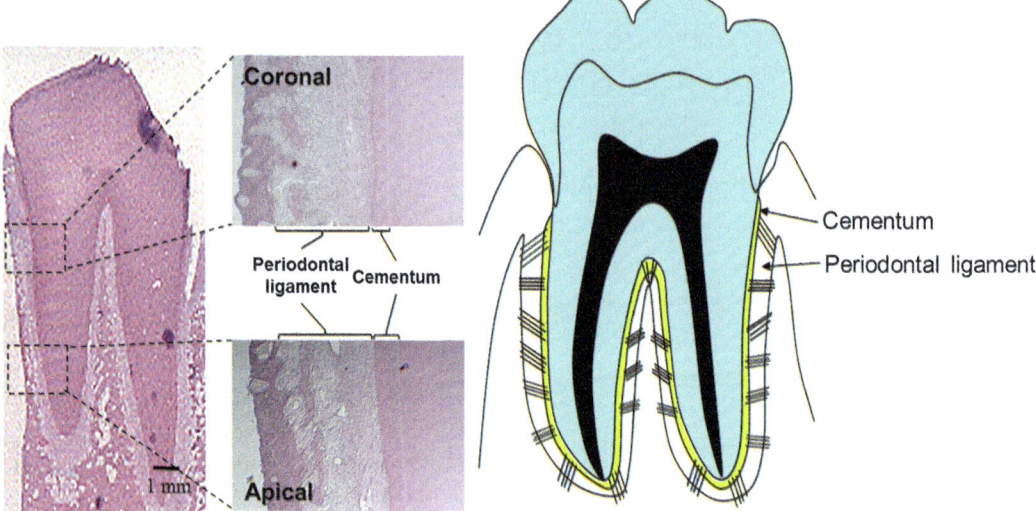

Fig. 5.1 Schematic illustration of periodontal tissues. Periodontal ligament (PDL) consists of different cell populations in various differentiation stages according to the position in PDL. Therefore, PDL plays an important role in the maintenance of periodontal tissues. Although cementum has many properties common to bone, there are distinct structural and functional differences between these two mineralized tissues: cementum has a limited remodeling potential; pathological cementum formation and defect cause structural disintegration and periodontal disease

mastication. Since a decrease of mechanical stress causes degenerative changes of periodontal tissues, mechanical stress has great influence on remodeling of the ligament and alveolar bone. Furthermore, in clinical orthodontics, when applying orthodontic force to tooth, bone resorption occurs on the compressive side and bone apposition also occurs on the tension side, followed by a widening of the PDL space and tooth migration toward the compressive side. Similar to osteocytes, mechanosensors in bone, PDL cells have been shown to directly respond to mechanical stimulation. Taken together, these clearly indicate that responses of PDL to mechanical stress are involved in its cell metabolism.

Cementum is a specialized mineralized tissue covering the root surface of the tooth and assists in anchoring teeth to surrounding alveolar bone, maintaining the structural stability and physiological function of the dentition [1]. Cementogenesis is initiated after root dentin formation and is regulated by interactions between Hertwig's epithelial root sheath and dental follicle mesenchymal cells [2]. Cementum has many properties common to bone and shows a marked similarity in biochemical composition. Fifty percent of cementum is composed of hydroxyapatite, while the remaining 50% is made up of collagen and a variety of proteoglycans and noncollagenous proteins, such as bone sialoprotein, osteocalcin, and osteopontin. However, there are distinct structural and functional differences between these two tissues: cementum has a limited remodeling potential, because cementoblasts are highly differentiated cells. Pathological cementum formation and defects cause structural disintegration and periodontal disease. Then, cementum regeneration can be lost as a result of disease or inflammation, such as periodontitis and root resorption.

Application of adequate mechanical stimulation to bone is essential for maintaining bone mass and strength. Mechanical stimuli have been reported to activate both osteoblasts and osteoclasts, resulting in the promotion of bone

Fig. 5.2 Schematic illustration of orthodontically induced root resorption. During orthodontic treatment, root resorption sometimes occurs because odontoclast is similar to osteoclast

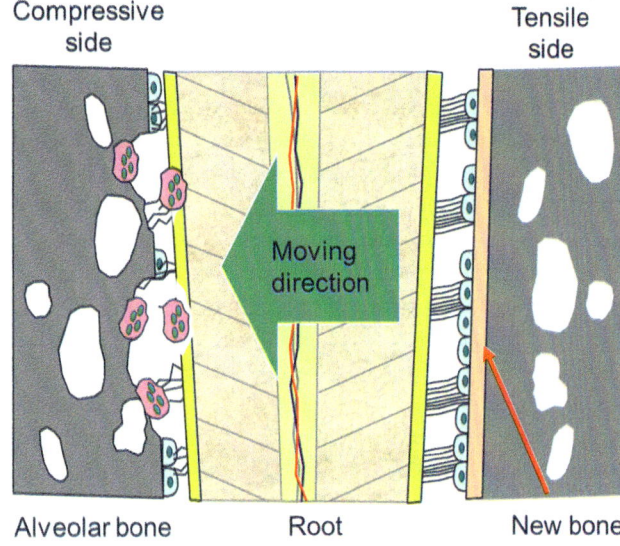

Fig. 5.3 Orthodontically induced root resorption. The fact is that orthodontic tooth movement directly causes an irreversible resorption of the root. Due to orthodontic tooth movement, the most severely resorbed teeth are maxillary central and lateral incisors, followed by the second premolars. Arrows indicate root resorption

Before treatment

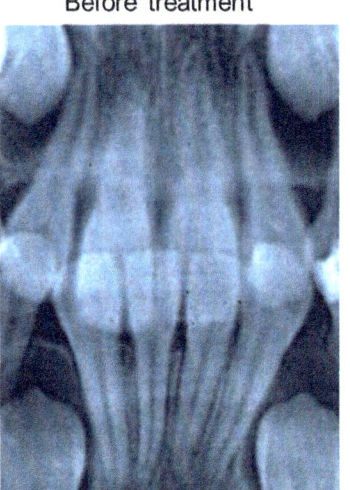

After treatment

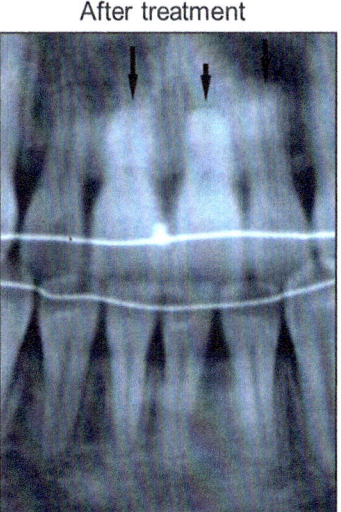

remodeling. During orthodontic treatment, root resorption sometimes occurs because odontoclast is similar to osteoclast (Fig. 5.2). Therefore, root resorption can be a relevant adverse outcome of orthodontic treatment. It is a fact that orthodontic tooth movement directly causes an irreversible resorption of the root (Fig. 5.3). The most severely resorbed teeth because of orthodontic tooth movement are maxillary central and lateral incisors, followed by the second premolars. A certain degree of root resorption occurs in most treatment cases, ranging from just a slight apical resorption to a complete tooth root loss [3, 4]. Root resorption during orthodontic treatment is a multifactorial event, and several biological and mechanical factors have been identified to increase its susceptibility; however, the exact mechanism still remains unclear [5, 6]. It is well accepted that the cementum layer covering the root surface plays a crucial role in preventing resorption during orthodontic tooth movement. In addition, the damaged areas are also repaired in part by cementoblasts lining the root surface. Cementoblast adhesion and activation and the subsequent root repair are assumed to be associated with temporospatial expression and maturation of various extracellular matrix proteins. Cementoblasts share many characteristics with osteoblasts, including similar molecular properties and the ability to promote mineralization [7]. Previous studies have shown that, as in bone, cementum metabolism is also controlled by mechanical stimulus. Unfortunately, therapies for protection against root resorption and/or for repairs of absorbed roots have been limited.

Repair of soft tissues injuries consists of three phases (inflammatory, proliferative, and remodeling phases), as with hard tissues healing process. It has been demonstrated both in the laboratory and in clinical trials that ultrasound can stimulate tissue repair and wound healing if correctly applied [8, 9]. It appears that exposure to ultrasound during the inflammatory phase of tissue repair can lead to an acceleration of this phase, which may eventually lead to an anti-inflammatory effect by LIPUS exposure [10, 11]. The second phase of healing is the "proliferative" stage. This is the stage at which cells migrate to the site of injury and start to divide, granulation tissue is formed, and fibroblasts begin to synthesize collagen. Ultrasound has been shown to enhance collagen synthesis by fibroblasts [12]. As a consequence, LIPUS may be a promising candidate of treatment remedy for periodontal diseases such as periodontitis and orthodontically induced root resorption.

5.2   In Vitro Studies

As described above, PDL cells possess stem cell properties, which play a key role in periodontal tissue regeneration. Like bone marrow stromal cells, PDL cells have the ability to give rise to mesoderm cell lineages, such as alveolar bone, cementum, and PDL for periodontal tissue regeneration [13, 14]. As the major aim of periodontal therapy is to prevent further attachment loss and

predictably restore the periodontal supporting structures, new bone formation is critical for maintaining the structural stability and physiological function of the dentition [1]. Therefore, to promote osteogenic differentiation of PDL cells during wound healing and regeneration is of great importance for treatment of periodontal diseases. In a previous study, it has been shown that cyclic stretch stimulation mediated PDL cells' differentiation, thus regulating the function of the PDL as a source of cementoblasts and osteoblasts through the EGF/EGF-R system [15]. In addition, it has been reported that LIPUS is effective in releasing fibroblast growth factors from a macrophage-like cell line [16]. Inubushi et al. [17] reported that LIPUS induced early cementoblastic differentiation of human immature cementoblasts from the PDL by promoting the formation of substrate and increasing alkaline phosphatase (ALP) activity, enabling the regeneration of periodontal tissue destroyed by periodontal disease and the acceleration of the repair of root resorption. Mostafa et al. [18] demonstrated that ALP and osteopontin expression were also induced in human gingival fibroblasts treated with LIPUS, confirming that after 3 weeks of 5 min/day exposure the osteogenic differentiation potential was enhanced. Recent studies also suggested that LIPUS promotes osteogenic differentiation of human PDL cells, which is associated with upregulation of Runx2 and integrin β1 [19] and activation of bone morphogenetic protein-smad signaling [20], which may thus provide therapeutic benefits in periodontal tissue regeneration. Therefore, it can be hypothesized that LIPUS might promote the differentiation of immature cementoblasts and PDL cells into mature cementoblasts and/or osteoblasts, leading to periodontal tissue regeneration and repair.

Using an immortalized mouse cementoblast cell line, OCCM-30, studies performed by our group showed that LIPUS upregulated the expression of several genes related to mineral metabolism [21] and enhanced PGE_2 production inducing cementoblastic differentiation and matrix mineralization through EP2/EP4 prostaglandin receptor pathway [22]. It was also shown in vitro that LIPUS impairs the lipopolysaccharide (LPS)-

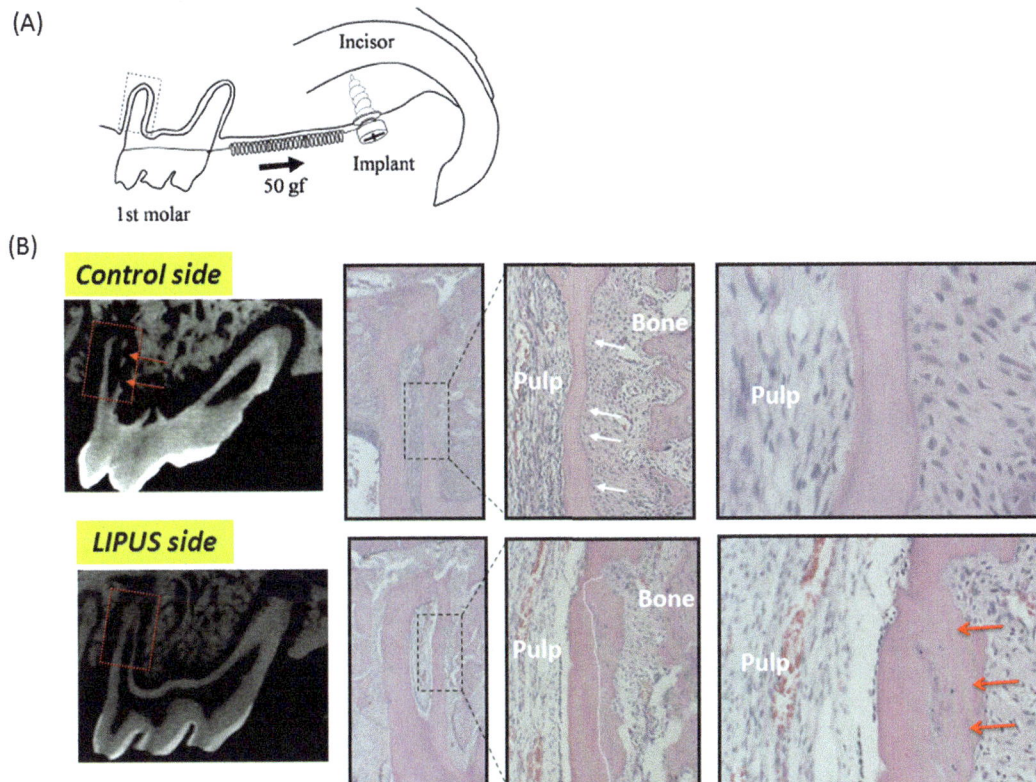

Fig. 5.4 (**a**) Schematic representation of the appliance for tooth movement. The axillary first molar was protracted using 50 gf activated Ni–Ti coil spring. (**b**) Micro-CT and histological observation. Representative histological sections (40x) of the upper first molar distobuccal root from 2-week time period stained with H.E. Resorption lacunae considerably occurred along the root in the control group, while in the LIPUS group root resorption was not obvious. White arrows indicate resorption lacunae. Red arrows indicate new bone apposition; white dotted line indicates border of root surface. (Modified from Inubushi et al. [26])

induced expression of tumor necrosis factor (TNF)-α mRNA in cementoblastic cells [23]. Moreover, LIPUS treatment inhibited the TNF-α-induced upregulation of *Rankl* mRNA [23]. Therefore, LIPUS may contribute to the reduction of the inflammatory reaction through impairment of the TNF-α signaling pathway. These indicate that LIPUS shows potential as a therapeutic tool to optimize the regenerative capacity of cementoblasts on periodontal diseases such as periodontitis and orthodontically induced root resorption.

5.3   In Vivo Studies

It has been reported that mechanical loading enhances the expression of phenotypic markers such as osteocalcin and bone sialoprotein in cementoblast in vivo; however, the expression was just moderately stimulated compared to osteoblasts [24]. Regarding ultrasound stimulation, a pioneer study published by El-Bialy et al. [25] showed that LIPUS prevented root resorption during experimental tooth movement in humans. Furthermore, in vivo study using an orthodontically induced root resorption model revealed that LIPUS exposure significantly reduced root resorption by the suppression of cementoclastogenesis during orthodontic tooth movement without interfering with tooth movement, suggestively by altering OPG/RANKL expression ratio [26] (Fig. 5.4). LIPUS induced the formation of a precementum layer, thicker cementum ,and reparative cellular cementum, resulting in significant reduction of the number and area of

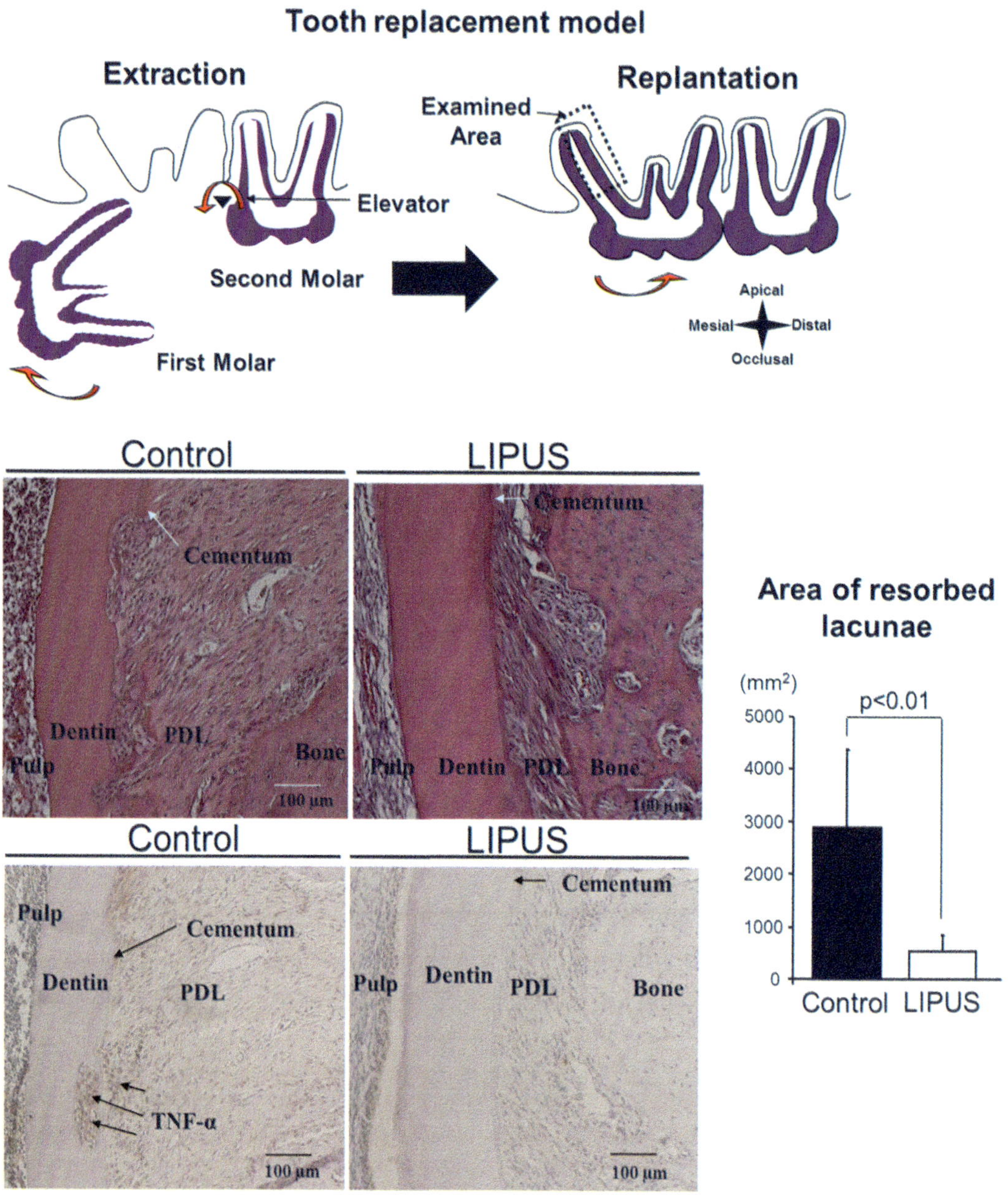

Tooth replacement model

Fig. 5.5 Schematic representation of an experimental model for extraction, replantation, and selection of the examined area. From histological findings of a replanted tooth, in the control group, substantial root resorption was observed on the distal side of the mesial root of the upper first molar 21 d after replantation. On the LIPUS-treated specimens, the development of severe root resorption lacunae was substantially prevented and cementum integrity could be observed along the root surface. From immunohistochemical staining, on the control specimen, positive staining of tumor necrosis factor-a (TNF-a) was evident and notably seen along the root resorption lacunae (arrows). On the LIPUS-treated specimens, however, positive staining of TNF-a was almost negligible after the 21-d treatment period. From histomorphometrical analysis, the area of resorption lacunae was significantly ($p < 0.01$) decreased by ultrasound therapy when compared with the untreated specimens (control). (Modified from Rego et al. [23])

orthodontically induced inflammatory root resorption [27]. Taking all together, it is anticipated that LIPUS can be a clinically effective therapy to prevent orthodontically induced root resorption in the future (See Chap. 11).

Apart from orthodontically induced root resorption, Rego et al. [23] assessed the inhibitory effect of a 21-day LIPUS application on root resorption using an experimental model of tooth replantation involving luxation and immediate replacement of maxillary first molars in rats (Fig. 5.5). The results showed that the area of root resorption lacunae was statistically decreased in LIPUS-treated sample. In addition, the expression of tumor necrosis factor (TNF)-α was not observed in LIPUS-treated sample as was evident in the control sample. This indicates that LIPUS has a potential as a therapeutic tool to optimize the regenerative potential of periodontal tissues on replanted teeth.

Recent studies have shown that LIPUS can enhance periodontal tissue repair and regeneration, especially if combined with the other treatment remedies for periodontal diseases such as guided tissue regeneration (GTR) [28–30]. This indicates achieving much better outcome of periodontal tissue repair and regeneration and shortening the periodontal tissue repair time by LIPUS exposure [28]. Furthermore, Ikai et al. [31] reported that the processes in regeneration of both cementum and alveolar bone were accelerated by LIPUS, leading to early periodontal wound healing and bone repair [31]. It is suggested that LIPUS could potentially enhance periodontal tissue repair and regeneration combined with GTR and provide therapeutic benefits in periodontal tissue regeneration.

References

1. Ten Cate AR. The periodontium: oral histology, development, structure and function. St Louis, MO: Mosby; 2003. p. 276–9.
2. Bosshardt DD, Schroeder HE. Cementogenesis reviewed: a comparison between human premolars and rodent molars. Anat Rec. 1996;245:267–92.
3. Hollender L, Ronneman A, Thilander B. Root resorption, marginal bone support and clinical crown length in orthodontically treated patients. Eur J Orthod. 1980;2:197–205.
4. Kurol J, Owman-Moll P, Lundgren D. Time related root resorption after application of a controlled continuous orthodontic force. Am J Orthod Dentofac Orthop. 1996;110:303–10.
5. Rita FN, David EW, James LG. Tooth resorption. Quint Int. 1999;30:9–25.
6. Sameshima GT, Sinclair PM. Predicting and preventing root resorption: Part II. Treatment factors. Am J Orthod Dentofac Orthop. 2001;119(5):511.
7. Matias MA, Li H, Young WG, Bartold PM. Immunohistochemical localization of extracellular matrix proteins in the periodontium during cementogenesis in the rat molar. Arch Oral Biol. 2003;48:709–16.
8. Dyson M, Pond JB, Joseph J, Warwick R. The stimulation of tissue regeneration by means of ultrasound. Clin Sci. 1968;35:273–85.
9. Dyson M. Therapeutic applications of ultrasound. In: Nyborg WL, Ziskin MC, editors. Biological effects of ultrasound. New York, NY: Churchill Livingstone; 1985. p. 121–33.
10. Iashchenko LV, Ostapiak ZN, Semenov VL. The humoral mechanisms of the action of ultrasound in inflammatory lung diseases (an experimental study). Vopr Kurortol Fizioter Lech Fiz Kult. 1994;2:20–2.
11. Mukai S, Ito H, Nakagawa Y, Akiyama H, Miyamoto M, Nakamura T. Transforming growth factor-β1 mediates the effects of low-intensity pulsed ultrasound in chondrocytes. Ultrasound Med Biol. 2005;31:1713–21.
12. Mortimer AJ, Dyson M. The effect of therapeutic ultrasound on calcium uptake in fibroblasts. Ultrasound Med Biol. 1988;14:499–506.
13. Washio K, Iwata T, Mizutani M, Ando T, Yamato M, Okano T, Ishikawa I. Assessment of cell sheets derived from human periodontal ligament cells: a pre-clinical study. Cell Tissue Res. 2010;341:397–404.
14. Yoshida T, Washio K, Iwata T, Okano T, Ishikawa I. Current status and future development of cell transplantation therapy for periodontal tissue regeneration. Int J Dent. 2012;2012:1–8.
15. Matsuda N, Yokoyama K, Takeshita S, Watanabe M. Role of epidermal growth factor and its receptor in mechanical stress-induced differentiation of human periodontal ligament cells in vitro. Arch Oral Biol. 1988;43:987–97.
16. Warden SJ, Favaloro JM, Bennell KL, McMeeken JM, Ng KW, Zajac JD, Wark JD. Low-intensity pulsed ultrasound stimulates a bone forming response in UMR-106 cells. Biochem Biophys Res Commun. 2001;286:443–50.
17. Inubushi T, Tanaka E, Rego EB, Kitagawa M, Kawazoe A, Ohta A, et al. Effects of ultrasound on the proliferation and differentiation of cementoblast lineage cells. J Periodontol. 2008;79:1984–90.
18. Mostafa NZ, Uludağ H, Dederich DN, Doschak MR, El-Bialy TH. Anabolic effects of low-intensity pulsed ultrasound on human gingival fibroblasts. Arch Oral Biol. 2009;54(8):743.

19. Hu B, Zhang Y, Zhou J, Li J, Deng F, Wang Z, Song J. Low-intensity pulsed ultrasound stimulation facilitates osteogenic differentiation of human periodontal ligament cells. PLoS One. 2014;9:e95168.

20. Yang Z, Ren L, Deng F, Wang Z, Song J. Low-intensity pulsed ultrasound induces osteogenic differentiation of human periodontal ligament cells through activation of bone morphogenetic protein-smad signaling. J Ultrasound Med. 2014;33:865–73.

21. Dalla-Bona DA, Tanaka E, Oka H, Yamano E, Kawai N, Miyauchi M, et al. Effects of ultrasound on cementoblast metabolism in vitro. Ultrasound Med Biol. 2006;32:943–8.

22. Rego EB, Inubushi T, Kawazoe A, Tanimoto K, Miyauchi M, Tanaka E, et al. Ultrasound stimulation induces PGE_2 synthesis promoting cementoblastic differentiation through EP2/EP4 receptor pathway. Ultrasound Med Biol. 2010;36:907–15.

23. Rego EB, Inubushi T, Miyauchi M, Kawazoe A, Tanaka E, Takata T, Tanne K. Ultrasound stimulation attenuates root resorption on rat replanted molars and impairs TNF-α signaling in vitro. J Periodont Res. 2011;46:648–54.

24. Norvell SM, Alvarez M, Bidwell JP, Pavalko FM. Fluid shear stress induces beta-catenin signaling in osteoblasts. Calcif Tissue Int. 2004;75:396–404.

25. El-Bialy T, El-Shamy I, Graber TM. Repair of orthodontically induced root resorption by ultrasound in humans. Am J Orthod Dentofac Orthop. 2004;126:186–93.

26. Inubushi T, Tanaka E, Rego EB, Ohtani J, Kawazoe A, Tanne K, et al. Low-intensity ultrasound stimulation inhibits resorption of the tooth root induced by experimental force application. Bone. 2013;53:497–506.

27. Al-Daghreer S, Doschak M, Sloan AJ, Major PW, Heo G, Scurtescu C, et al. Effect of low-intensity pulsed ultrasound on orthodontically induced root resorption in beagle dogs. Ultrasound Med Biol. 2014;40:1187–96.

28. Gu XQ, Li YM, Guo J, Zhang LH, Li D, Gai XD. Effect of low intensity pulsed ultrasound on repairing the periodontal bone of Beagle canines. Asian Pac J Trop Med. 2014;7:325–8.

29. Wang Y, Chai Z, Zhang Y, Deng F, Wang Z, Song J. Influence of low-intensity pulsed ultrasound on osteogenic tissue regeneration in a periodontal injury model: X-ray image alterations assessed by micro-computed tomography. Ultrasonics. 2014;54:1581–4.

30. Zheng H, Lu L, Song JL, Deng F, Wang ZB. Low intensity pulsed ultrasound combined with guided tissue regeneration for promoting the repair of defect at canines periodontal fenestration in Beagle dogs. Zhonghua Kou Qiang Yi Xue Za Zhi. 2011;46:431–6.

31. Ikai H, Tamura T, Watanabe T, Itou M, Sugaya A, Iwabuchi S, et al. Low-intensity pulsed ultrasound accelerates periodontal wound healing after flap surgery. J Periodontal Res. 2008;43:212–6.

Application of LIPUS to the Temporomandibular Joint

Eiji Tanaka, Tatsuya Nakamura, Minami Sato, Harmanpreet Kaur, and Tarek El-Bialy

Abstract

The most common joint pathology affecting the temporomandibular joint (TMJ) is degenerative joint disease, also known as osteoarthritis (OA). TMJ-OA is characterized by mandibular condylar cartilage degradation due to mechanical overloading. Rheumatoid arthritis (RA) is also a systemic, chronic inflammatory disease of the TMJ with cartilage destruction and infiltration of inflammatory cells into synovial tissue. Since the fibrocartilage covering both the TMJ condyle and articular eminence is avascular, these fibrocartilage cells have limited ability to self-repair. Therefore, once the breakdown in the joint starts, TMJ-OA and TMJ-RA can be crippling, leading to a variety of morphological and functional deformities. From in vitro and in vivo studies, low-intensity pulsed ultrasound (LIPUS) downregulates COX-2 and PGE_2 expression, upregulates HAS2 and HAS3 expression, and suppresses the proliferation and growth in IL-1-β-stimulated synovial membrane cells and reduces COX-2 expression and synovial hyperplasia in RA joints. These results are indicative of distinct anabolic effect of LIPUS application that enhances the TMJ metabolism and regeneration. In conclusion, LIPUS may be a medical treatment option for degenerative joint diseases such as RA and OA.

E. Tanaka (✉)
Department of Orthodontics and Dentofacial Orthopedics, Institute of Biomedical Sciences, Tokushima University Graduate School, Tokushima, Japan

Department of Orthodontics, King Abdulaziz University, Jeddah, Saudi Arabia
e-mail: etanaka@tokushima-u.ac.jp

T. Nakamura
Kawakami Orthodontic Clinic, Takamatsu, Japan

M. Sato
Department of Orthodontics and Dentofacial Orthopedics, Institute of Biomedical Sciences, Tokushima University Graduate School, Tokushima, Japan

H. Kaur
Department of Dentistry, University of Alberta, Edmonton, Canada

T. El-Bialy
Dentistry/Orthodontics and Biomedical Engineering, University of Alberta, Edmonton, Alberta, Canada

6.1 Introduction

Synovial joints allow various degrees of relative motion of the bones produced by surrounding muscle forces [1]. The bone ends come together within a fibrous joint capsule. The inner lining of this joint capsule is a metabolically active tissue, known as the synovium. The ends of the bones are covered by a thin and highly deformable layer of dense connective tissue known as articular cartilage [2]. Ligaments, tendons, and other soft tissues inside and outside the joint cavity give stability to the joint and maintain the proper

© Springer International Publishing AG, part of Springer Nature 2018
T. El-Bialy et al. (eds.), *Therapeutic Ultrasound in Dentistry*,
https://doi.org/10.1007/978-3-319-66323-4_6

Fig. 6.1 Anatomy of the temporomandibular joint (TMJ)

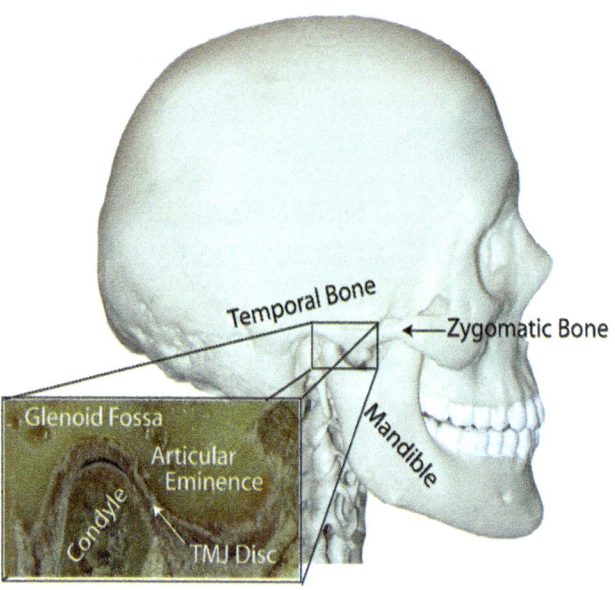

alignment of the articulating bone ends during motion [2]. Daily activity accompanies joint motion, resulting in joint loads. The temporomandibular joint (TMJ), a diarthrodial synovial joint, enables large relative movements between the temporal bone and the mandibular condyle [3, 4] (Fig. 6.1). The integrity of the joint is maintained by a fibrous capsule with its intrinsic ligamentous thickenings and extrinsically by accessory ligaments. Both of these ligaments act as restraints to movement at the extremes of mandibular range of motion and thus have limited influence on the mechanics of normal symmetrical function (Fig. 6.2). Within the joint, the articular surfaces of the condyle and articular eminence are each covered by a thin fibrocartilaginous layer having a very low coefficient of friction [5] (Fig. 6.3). A dense fibrocartilaginous articular disc is located between the bones in each TMJ. The articular disc divides the joint cavity into two compartments (superior and inferior) and is a structure with an important functional role. The disc provides a largely passive movable articular surface accommodating the translatory movement made by the condyle. Since the fibrocartilage covering both the mandibular condyle and articular eminence is avascular and the disc is composed of basically the same avascular

tissue, intra-articular synovial fluid provides nourishment to these fibrocartilaginous cells which also have limited ability to self-repair [6–8]. Histologically, mandibular condylar cartilage (MCC) is divided into four layers based on the distribution of collagen I, II, and X. Superficial layer adjacent to the joint cavity is the articular or fibrous layer. Superficial zone protein (SZP) is expressed in this layer which acts as a lubricant for the joint activity. There is no cellular differentiation in this zone as this layer mainly functions as a protective covering for the underlying layers [9, 10]. Next layer is the proliferative or polymorphic zone and is composed of irregular polygonal cells in the upper layer while lower layer has flattened cells with their long axis parallel to the articular layer. Cells in this layer are actively proliferating and express parathyroid hormone-related protein (PTHrP) and SRY-box containing gene 9 (SOX9). These cells have multilineage potential to differentiate into chondroblasts, osteoblasts, or fat progenitor cells depending on the presence of mechanical load [11]. The third layer is the chondrocyte cell layer in which there is a change in cellular morphology from flattened to spherical cells. This layer shows increased deposition of collagen, proteoglycans, and glycosaminoglycans (GAGs) [12]. Indian

Closing position   **Open position**

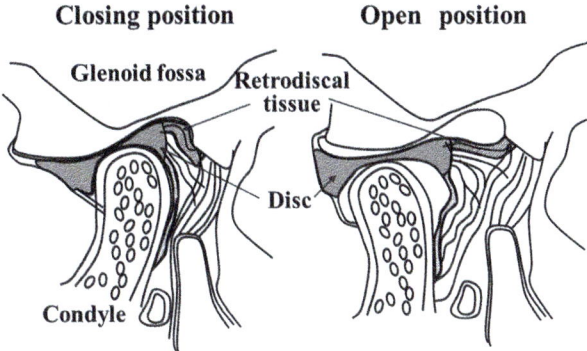

Fig. 6.2 Sagittal views of the TMJ. The TMJ consists of the bone components (mandibular condyle and articular eminence) and soft tissues (condylar cartilage, fossa cartilage, joint capsule, articular disc, and retrodiscal tissue). In the healthy joint, the articular disc moves forward and downward when the mandibular condyle moves along the posterior slope of the articular eminence (mouth opening). Both at closing and opening positions, the disc is located between the two bone components. The articular surfaces are covered with thin fibrous layers. Synovial fluid inside the joints acts as a lubricant during movement

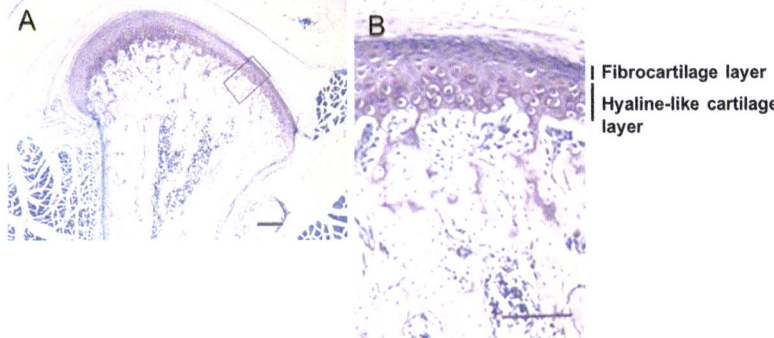

Fig. 6.3 Photomicrographs of the TMJ and the articular cartilage layer. Cartilage layers of condyle in 16-week-old male rats were visualized by toluidine blue staining. Bar indicates 200 mm (**a**) and 100 mm (**b**)

hedgehog (Ihh) is expressed in a pre-hypertrophic layer that regulates PTHrP level by a negative feedback loop. In the fourth layer, which is the hypertrophic cell layer, the chondrocytes increase in volume and become hypertrophic. There is a transition from collagen II to collagen X. With this, the degradation of cartilage begins, a preliminary stage of endochondral ossification [13]. Chondrocyte hypertrophic differentiation is believed to be regulated by Runt-related transcription factor 2 (RUNX2), an important transcription factor for osteoblast differentiation [14]. RUNX2 positively controls Ihh expression by activating its promoter gene and hence regulating PTHrP expression [15].

MCC has the capability to grow in multi-direction; hence, it has a unique characteristic to adapt to the external stimuli throughout life [16]. Mechanical stress is also an important factor that differentiates the progenitor cells in the superficial layer of MCC to either chondroblasts or osteoblasts as these cells have shown to express both SOX and RUNX2 [17]. Increased mechanical loading on MCC has shown to increase cell proliferation and increased collagen II synthesis [18, 19]. Mechanical loading initiates specific biomechanical responses in the chondrocytes. This distinctive characteristic is the fundamental rationale for therapies with different types of orthopedic appliances also known as functional appliances.

Disturbance in the form of mutation or deletion of any factor besides mechanical loading severely affects MCC growth and development. Deficient mandible can be present as an isolated condition or in association with over 450 syndromic conditions. Congenital problems include hemifacial microsomia, Treacher Collin syndrome, and Pierre Robin syndrome that affect the mandibular development, while Class II malocclusion is also characterized by underdeveloped mandible.

The synovial membrane contains specialized cell types with phagocytic and immunologic capacity and produces synovial fluid. Synovial fluid is a viscous gel and contains mostly water and acts as a lubricant in joints as well as a vehicle for nutrients as it passes through the surfaces of articular cartilage layers [5, 20–22]. Most of the other synovial joints are discless joints and the articular cartilage is hyaline cartilage. The fibrocartilaginous nature of the TMJ disc and articular cartilage along with the lubrication function of the intra-articular synovial fluid allow the cartilaginous structures of the TMJ to conform under function and ensure that loads are absorbed and spread over larger contact areas [23–26]. Hyaluronan (HA), 0.14–0.36% of synovial fluid in normal subjects [27], is one of the principal components determining the rheological properties of synovial fluid [28]. Furthermore, it has been suggested that mechanical stimuli play a crucial role in regulating HA metabolism, and HA synthesis by synovial membrane cells is affected by mechanical stimuli [29]. Up to present, three kinds of HA synthase (HAS1, HAS2, and HAS3) have been reported [30]. HAS1 and HAS2 polymerize HA chains of similar lengths (up to 2×10^3 kDa), whereas HAS3 produces shorter chains (200–300 kDa) [30]. In synovial fluid, HA with high molecular weight released by type B synovial membrane cells is generally believed to be essential for lubrication of joints by reducing friction [31]. Hyaluronidase (HYAL) has been known to play a crucial role in HA catabolism in joints [32]. With the possible exception of HYAL4 and HYALP1, all other HYALs have an ability to degrade HA [33]. HYAL2 degrades high-molecular-weight HA into small fragments of HA with a molecular weight of approximately 20 kDa [33]. Among these HYALs, HYAL1 and HYAL2 are detected in synovial membrane, and HYAL activity was highly detected in the synovial fluid obtained from rheumatoid arthritis (RA) patients [34]. Recently, we evaluated the effects of cyclic tensile load on the expression and activity of HYAL in synovial membrane cells and suggested that increased HA by mechanical stimuli affects HA catabolism in synovial fluid [29]. TMJ disorders (TMDs) are characterized by intra-articular morphologic abnormalities, such as traumatic, degenerative, and/or inflammatory arthritic pathology and developmental, congenital, and neoplastic processes. A review of 18 epidemiologic studies published in the 1980s reported prevalence rates ranging from 16 to 59% for reported symptoms and 33–86% for clinical signs [35], although 3–7% of the adult population have sought care for TMD-related pain and dysfunction [36]. It has been observed that up to 70% of patients with TMDs suffer from displacement of the articular disc, coined internal derangement of the TMJ (TMJ-ID) [37]. In particular, the most common joint pathology affecting the TMJ is degenerative joint disease, also known as osteoarthrosis or osteoarthritis (OA). TMJ-OA is characterized by mandibular condylar cartilage degradation due to mechanical overloading [38]. Mechanical overloading of the mandibular condylar cartilage induces the expression of IL-1β [39], an inflammatory cytokine closely related to the progression of TMJ-OA [40–42] (Fig. 6.4). Thus, a large amount of IL-1β has been detected in the synovial fluid of patients with TMJ-OA [43]. Since the fibrocartilage covering both the TMJ condyle and articular eminence is avascular, these fibrocartilage cells have limited ability to self-repair [44, 45]. Therefore, once the breakdown in the joint starts, TMJ-OA can be crippling, leading to a variety of morphological and functional deformities. This suggests the importance of suppression of cartilage degradation during the early stage of TMJ-OA.

RA is a systemic, chronic inflammatory disease of synovial joints including the TMJ that is characterized by synovial hyperplasia, cartilage destruction, and infiltration of inflammatory cells into synovial tissue [46]. It is widely

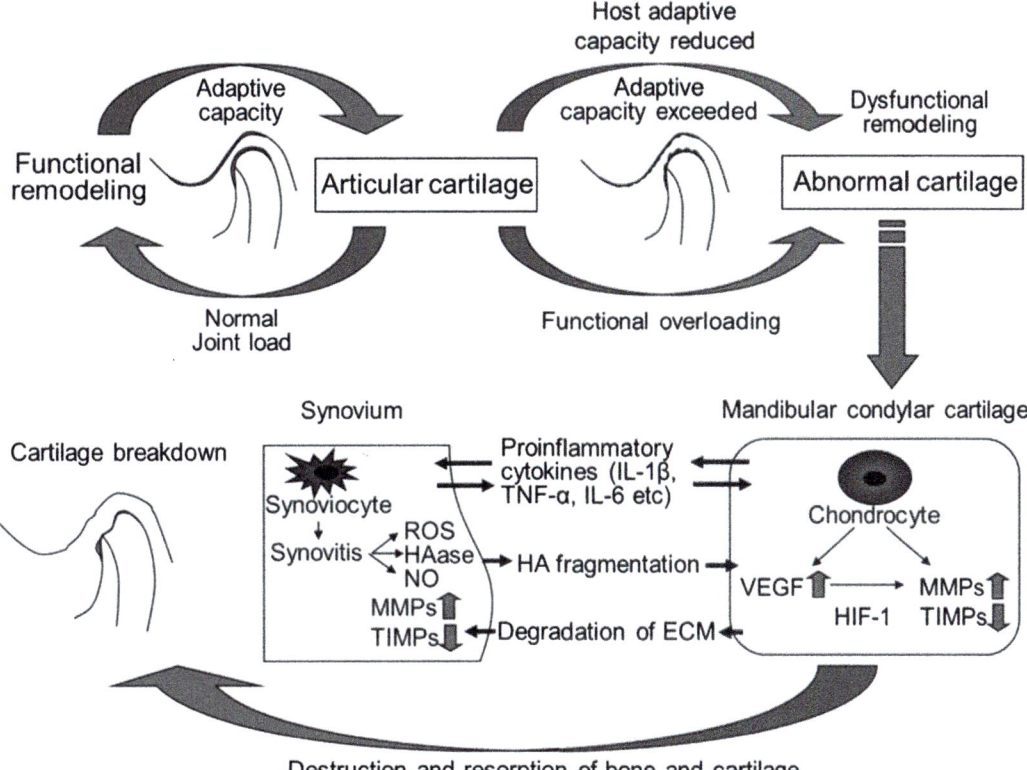

Fig. 6.4 Schematic illustrations of the concept of mandibular condylar cartilage degradation. Functional overloading can facilitate hypoxia in the TMJ which mediates the destructive processes associated with osteoarthrosis as an autocrine factor. VEGF induction in OA-cartilage by functional overloading is linked to activation of the HIF-1, leading to hypoxia in the joint tissue. Furthermore, VEGF regulates the production of MMPs and TIMPs which are among the effectors of extracellular matrix remodeling. Overloading also causes collapse of joint lubrication as a result of the HA degradation by free radicals. The regulation of HA production is controlled by various pro-inflammatory cytokines. (Modified from Tanaka et al. [22])

accepted that synovitis is associated with clinical symptoms and reflects joint degradation in RA [47], and several studies have focused attention on synovial hyperplasia [48]. Synovial hyperplasia is a major pathophysiologic feature of RA and appears to be associated with pro-inflammatory cytokines, notably TNF-α and IL-1β [47]. Therefore, the importance of synovitis in the pathophysiology of RA has been increasingly recognized, particularly in early stages of the disease. Furthermore, synovial fibroblasts in the synovial intimal lining play a key role in producing cytokines and proteases [49]. Since targeting synovial fibroblasts may improve clinical outcomes in inflammatory arthritis, it is thought that the control of proliferation and viability of synovial fibroblasts is an important consideration for treatment strategies.

6.2 In Vitro Studies

Previously, LIPUS has been reported to affect cartilage matrix metabolism through integrin β1, a possible cell surface receptor for LIPUS in chondrocytes [50]. However, chondrocytes derived from hyaline cartilages were used in these studies. Therefore, study by Iwabuchi et al. [51] is the first attempt to investigate the effects of LIPUS on mandibular condylar chondrocytes metabolism. Iwabuchi et al. [51] elucidated the effect of LIPUS on COX-2 expression and related mechanisms by using cultured articular chondrocytes derived from porcine mandibular condyles after treatment with IL-1β. TMJs were obtained from female pigs aged 6–9 months. Mandibular condylar cartilage was carefully dissected from the mandible, and the condylar cartilage pieces were digested in Dulbecco's modified Eagle medium (DMEM). Isolated chondrocytes were cultured and received LIPUS. An ultrasound exposure assembly, BR-Sonic Pro (ITO Co., Tokyo, Japan), was employed in a series of experiments. LIPUS was exposed immediately after the addition of 0 or 10 ng/ml IL-1β. The probe of this system consists of a 9.6-cm^2 circular surface transducer area. The sound head of this device has an average beam nonuniformity ratio (BNR) of 3.1–3.5:1 and an effective radiating area (ERA) of 4.5 cm^2 (46.8%). A pulsed ultrasound signal was transmitted at a frequency of 3 MHz, with a spatial average temporal average intensity of 30 mW/cm^2, and pulsed at 20% (2 ms on and 8 ms off) for 20 min. Control samples were also subjected to the same operations under the same conditions without LIPUS stimulation. As a result, COX-2 mRNA level was upregulated by the treatment with IL-1β and was

suppressed significantly by LIPUS exposure. Furthermore, LIPUS enhanced gene expression and phosphorylation of integrin β, and it inhibited the expression of p-ERK1/2. It was concluded that LIPUS exposure inhibited IL-1β-induced COX-2 expression through the integrin β1 receptor followed by the phosphorylation of ERK1/2 (Fig. 6.5). This indicates that LIPUS is suggested to be a potential candidate as a preventive and auxiliary treatment to suppress the degradation of articular chondrocytes in TMJ-OA, leading to tissue engineering in the mandibular condylar cartilage. In this line, El-Bialy et al. [52] reported that LIPUS enhanced chondrogenic and osteogenic differentiation of bone marrow stromal cells, resulting in ultrasound-assisted tissue-engineered mandibular condyles in vivo.

As described above, the HA metabolism would be affected by several pro-inflammatory cytokines, and relatively high concentration of TNF-α and IL-1β has been detected in the synovial fluid obtained from patients with OA [53] but not from healthy joints. IL-1β induced the accumulation of low-molecular-weight HA in cultured synovial membrane cells derived from OA and RA patients [54]. In human lung fibroblasts, IL-1β also accumulated low-molecular-weight HA, whereas TNF-α induced the accumulation

Fig. 6.5 Schematic illustration of possible signaling activated by LIPUS exposure. The mechanisms of repression of excessive COX-2 production caused by LIPUS may be due to the repression of ERK 1/2

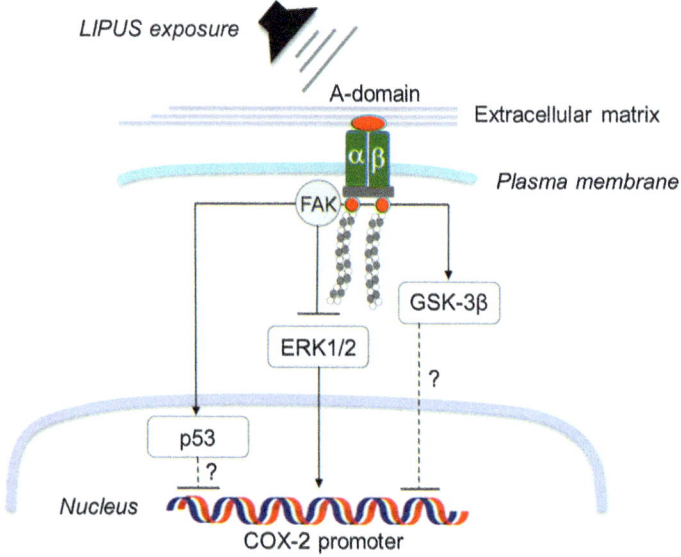

of high-molecular-weight HA [55]. Nakamura et al. [56] examined the effects of LIPUS exposure on metabolism of hyaluronan (HA) in synovial membrane cells stimulated by IL-1β. A LIPUS exposure system which was a modification of the clinical device (BR sonic-pro, ITO Co., Tokyo, Japan) was employed. This system consisted of a 9.6-cm^2 circular surface transducer and a culture flask. The beam nonuniformity ratio, the ratio between peak amplitude and the average amplitude of US beam across the effective radiating area (ERA), was 3.2–3.6, and ERA was 90%. A pulsed US signal was transmitted at a frequency = 3 MHz with a spatial-average intensity = 30 mW/cm^2 and pulsed 1:4 (2 ms on and 8 ms off). They showed that gene levels of HAS2 and HAS3 in IL-1β-stimulated cells were upregulated significantly by LIPUS and that HYAL2 mRNA was upregulated by the treatment with IL-1β while downregulated significantly following LIPUS exposure. Furthermore, IL-1β stimulation enhanced COX-2 and PGE$_2$ expression as compared to the untreated control, and IL-1β-induced COX-2 and PGE$_2$ expression was inhibited by LIPUS. These results suggest that LIPUS downregulates COX-2 and PGE$_2$ expression and upregulates HAS2 and HAS3 expression in IL-1β-stimulated synovial membrane cells, leading to promotion of anti-inflammatory system. Taken together, LIPUS might enhance synthesis of high-molecular-weight HA, indicating anti-inflammatory response.

With respect to the molecular mechanisms by which LIPUS suppresses synovial hyperplasia and synovial cell proliferation, it is very probable that LIPUS transmits signals into the cell via an integrin that acts as a mechanoreceptor on the cell membrane [57]. When LIPUS is transmitted to integrin molecules, this promotes the attachment of various focal adhesion adaptor proteins. FAK is in turn phosphorylated as a result of LIPUS exposure initiating this signal transduction. Sato et al. [44] showed that LIPUS induced a significant upregulation of phosphorylated FAK in the synovial cells and also that FAK phosphorylation inhibition led to significant downregulation of MAPK phosphorylation. Activation of integrins and the downstream signaling pathway has also

been reported based on an in vitro study of LIPUS using human skin fibroblasts [58]. Integrins act as a link between extracellular matrix, cytoskeletal proteins, and actin filaments, and Hsu et al. [59] reported treatment with anti-Integrin β1 and β3 antibodies or transfection with siRNA against Integrin β1 and β3 antagonized the potentiating action of LIPUS stimulation on COX-2 expression, indicating that Integrin β1 and β3 are very important to mediate the action of LIPUS in chondrocytes. Furthermore, it is reported that LIPUS exposure to cementoblasts mediated cell metabolism through MAPK pathway because LIPUS enhanced the protein expression of ERK1/2 and also based on the evidence that MEK1/2 inhibitor treatment suppressed the upregulation of Cox-2 mRNA expression induced by LIPUS [60]. The integrin/Ras/MAPK pathway is considered a general pathway involved in cell proliferation. Considering these findings, the bioeffect of LIPUS exposure to synovial cells might be promoted via integrin/FAK/MAPK pathway particularly (Fig. 6.6).

6.3 In Vivo Studies

El-Bialy et al. [61] firstly evaluated the effect of LIPUS on condylar and mandibular growth in the rabbit model with functional appliance and demonstrated that the daily use of LIPUS for 4 weeks stimulates mandibular condylar growth and increases the mandibular condylar, ramal, and total mandibular heights in growing rabbits. This indicates that LIPUS accelerates condylar and mandibular growth during orthopedic treatment. Oyonarte et al. [62] also investigated the morphological effects of LIPUS stimulation on the mandibular condyles of growing rats and demonstrated that LIPUS application may affect mandibular growth pattern in rats acting at the cartilage and bone level. They also indicated that the effect of LIPUS on the growing condyle is expressed through a variation in trabecular shape and perimeter. Furthermore, recent study by Oyonarte et al. [63] showed that LIPUS and mesenchymal stem cell (MSC) application to the TMJ region of growing rats favored transverse

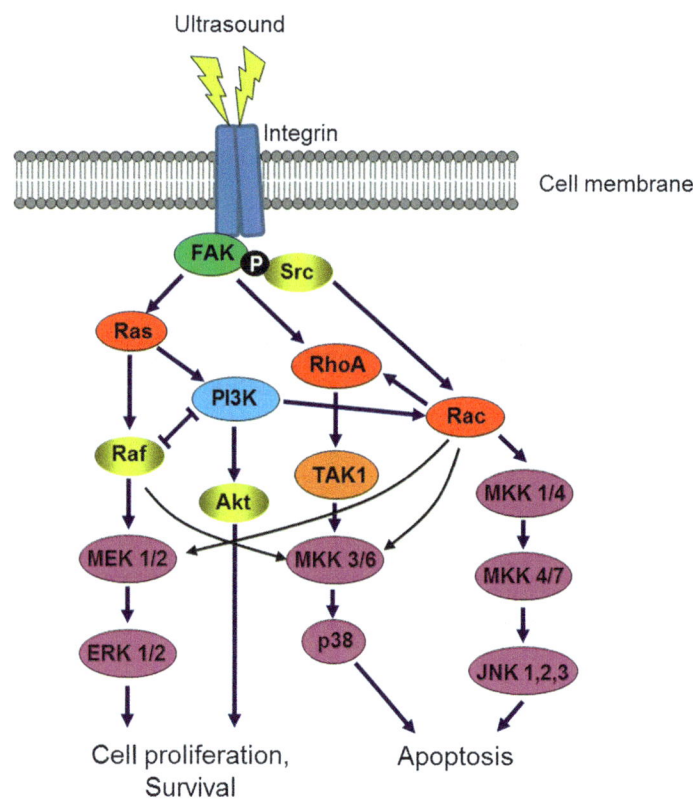

Fig. 6.6 Schematic illustration of mechanisms of signal transduction pathways enhanced by LIPUS. LIPUS may regulate synovial cell metabolism via integrin/FAK/MAPK pathway particularly. (Modified from Sato et al. [44])

condylar growth, while LIPUS application alone may enhance sagittal condylar development. These studies may give an insight regarding the utility of LIPUS as a novel treatment tool for patients with mandibular growth deficient. There has been some evidence in the literature that the effect of LIPUS on bone formation is dose dependent [63–66]. Kaur et al. [67] investigated the effect of LIPUS at two treatment durations—20 and 40 min along with functional appliances on the mandibular condylar growth in the growing rats. After 4 weeks, 20 min LIPUS application either alone or in combination with functional appliance showed a significant increase in mandibular condylar length and increased cell number and layer width of proliferative and hypertrophic layer. In addition, Micro-CT analysis demonstrated a significant increase in trabecular bone micro-architecture and bone mineral density as compared to 40 min LIPUS application. Furthermore, Kaur et al. [68] showed increased

mandibular condylar growth in either bFGF pDNA gene therapy or LIPUS groups compared to the combined group (bFGF pDNA + LIPUS) that showed only increased bone volume fraction. They also concluded that that there is an additive effect of bFGF + LIPUS on the mandibular growth.

Nakamura et al. [69] conducted in vivo study to examine the effectiveness of LIPUS treatment of synovitis in the knee joints of MRL/*lpr* mice, naturally induced RA animal model. A LIPUS exposure system was used that was modified from the clinical device (BR sonic-pro, ITO Co., Tokyo, Japan). This system consisted of a 4.5 cm^2 circular surface transducer and a culture flask. The beam nonuniformity ratio, which is defined as the ratio between the peak amplitude and the average amplitude of ultrasound beam across the effective radiating area (ERA), was 3.2–3.6. The ERA was 90%. A pulsed ultrasound signal was transmitted at a frequency of 3 MHz with a

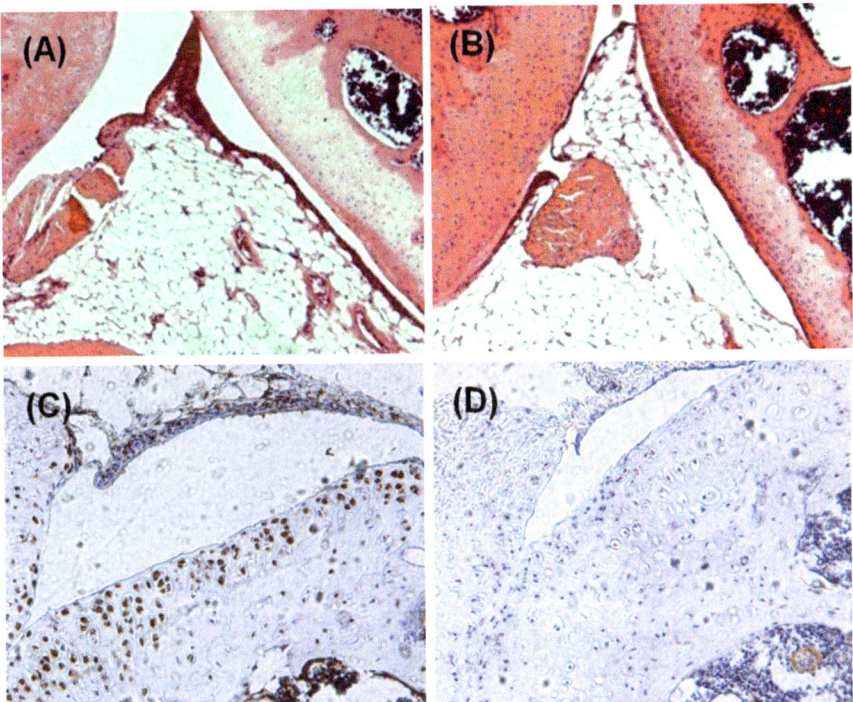

Fig. 6.7 Histological examination in the knee joints from MRL/lpr mice. The control side joint reveals proliferation of synovial cells and inflammatory cell infiltration (**a**), while the joint treated with LIPUS has relatively mild hyperplasia (**b**). From immunohistochemical staining of Cox-2 in the knee joints, an abundant number of Cox-2- positive cells are detected in the control joints that did not receive LIPUS exposure (**c**). Cox-2-positive cells are predominantly located in regions of synovium and cartilage. In contrast, Cox-2-positive cells in the knee joints treated with LIPUS are markedly decreased compared to the control joints (**d**). (Modified from Nakamura et al. [69])

spatial-average intensity of 30 mW/cm^2 and pulsed 1:4 (2 ms on and 8 ms off). As a result, histological lesions of RA were significantly reduced in the joints treated with LIPUS for 3 weeks (Fig. 6.7). COX-2-positive cells in the knee joints treated with LIPUS were markedly decreased compared to the control joints (Fig. 6.7). Therefore, the inhibition of COX-2 by LIPUS may play an important role in the suppression of inflammation. It can be hypothesized that the inhibition of COX-2 expression by LIPUS exposure inhibits cell proliferation in synovial tissue as a secondary effect. Considering these findings, LIPUS stimulation may also be a better candidate as medical remedy to treat inflammatory joint diseases accompanied with HA degradation in synovial fluid, such as synovitis.

6.4   Conclusions

LIPUS downregulates COX-2 and PGE$_2$ expression, upregulates HAS2 and HAS3 expression, and suppresses the proliferation and growth in IL-1β-stimulated synovial membrane cells in vitro and reduces COX-2 expression and synovial hyperplasia in RA joints in vivo. Collectively, these results are indicative of distinct anabolic effect of LIPUS application that enhances the TMJ metabolism and regeneration. Furthermore, LIPUS exposure inhibited IL-1-β-induced COX-2 expression through the integrin β1 receptor followed by the phosphorylation of ERK 1/2. Taken together, LIPUS may be a medical treatment option for degenerative joint diseases, such as rheumatoid arthritis and osteoarthritis in addition to treatment of deficient mandible where it can reduce the treatment duration when used synergistically with functional appliance.

References

1. Widegren U, Wretman C, Lionikas A, Hedin G, Henriksson J. Influence of exercise intensity on ERK/MAP kinase signalling in human skeletal muscle. Pflugers Arch. 2000;441:317–22.
2. Warwick R, Williams PL. Gray's anatomy. Philadelphia, PA: Saunders Co.; 1973.
3. Gray RJM, Davies SJ, Quayle AA. Temporomandibular disorders: a clinical approach. London: British Dental Association; 1995.
4. Rees LA. The structure and function of the mandibular joint. Br Dent J. 1954;96:125–33.
5. Tanaka E, Kawai N, Tanaka M, Todoh M, van Eijden T, Hanaoka K, et al. The Frictional coefficient of the temporomandibular joint and its dependency on the magnitude and duration of joint loading. J Dent Res. 2004;83:404–7.
6. Aoyama J, Tanaka E, Miyauchi M, Takata T, Hanaoka K, Hattori Y, et al. Immunolocalization of vascular endothelial growth factor in rat condylar cartilage during postnatal development. Histochem Cell Biol. 2004;122:35–40.
7. Fujisawa T, Kuboki T, Kasai T, Sonoyama W, Kajima S, Uehara J, et al. A repetitive steady mouth opening induced an osteoarthritis-like lesion in the rabbit temporomandibular joint. J Dent Res. 2003;82:731–5.
8. Tanaka E, Aoyama J, Miyauchi M, Takata T, Hanaoka K, Iwabe T, et al. Vascular endothelial growth factor plays an important autocrine/paracrine role in the progression of osteoarthritis. Histochem Cell Biol. 2005;123:275–81.
9. Luder HU, Leblond CP, von der Mark K. Cellular stages in cartilage formation as revealed by morphometry, radioautography and type II collagen immunostaining of the mandibular condyle from weanling rats. Am J Anat. 1988;182:197–214.
10. Ohno S, Schmid T, Tanne Y, Kamiya T, Honda K, Nakahara MO, et al. Expression of superficial zone protein in mandibular condyle cartilage. Osteoarthr Cart. 2006;14:807–13.
11. Mizoguchi I, Toriya N, Nakao Y. Growth of the mandible and biological characteristics of the mandibular condylar cartilage. Jpn Dent Sci Rev. 2013;49:139–50.
12. Fukada K, Shibata S, Suzuki S, Ohya K, Kuroda T. In situ hybridisation study of type I, II, X collagens and aggrecan mRNAs in the developing condylar cartilage of fetal mouse mandible. J Anat. 1999;195:321–9.
13. Shen G, Rabie ABM, Zhao ZH, Kaluarachchi K. Forward deviation of the mandibular condyle enhances endochondral ossification of condylar cartilage indicated by increased expression of type X collagen. Arch Oral Biol. 2006;51:315–24.
14. Park JH, Park BH, Kim HK, Park TS, Baek HS. Hypoxia decreases Runx2/Cbfa1 expression in human osteoblast-like cells. Mol Cell Endocrinol. 2002;192:197–203.
15. Hartmann C, Tabin CJ. Dual roles of Wnt signaling during chondrogenesis in the chicken limb. Development. 2000;127:3141–59.
16. Rabie ABM, Hägg U. Factors regulating mandibular condylar growth. Am J Orthod Dentofac Orthop. 2002;122:401–9.
17. Glineburg RW, Laskin DM, Blaustein DI. The effects of immobilization on the primate temporomandibular joint: a histologic and histochemical study. J Oral Maxillofac Surg. 1982;40:3–8.
18. Ghafari J, Degroote C. Condylar cartilage response to continuous mandibular displacement in the rat. Angle Orthod. 1986;5:49–57.
19. Nakao Y, Nagasaka MK, Toriya N, Arakawa T, Kashio H, Takuma T, Mizoguchi I. Proteoglycan expression is influenced by mechanical load in TMJ discs. J Dent Res. 2015;94:93–100.
20. Linn FC. Lubrication of animal joints—I. The arthrotripsometer. J Bone Joint Surg. 1967;49-A:1079–98.
21. Mabuchi K, Obara T, Ikegami K, Yamaguchi T, Kanayama T. Molecular weight independence of the effect of additive hyaluronic acid on the lubricating characteristics in synovial joints with experimental deterioration. Clin Biomech. 1999;14:352–6.
22. Tanaka E, Detamore MS, Mercuri LG. Degenerative disorders of the temporomandibular joint: etiology, diagnosis, and treatment. J Dent Res. 2008;87:296–307.
23. Nitzan DW. The process of lubrication impairment and its involvement in temporomandibular joint disc displacement: a theoretical concept. J Oral Maxillofac Surg. 2001;59:36–45.
24. Scapino RP, Canham PB, Finlay HM, Mills DK. The behaviour of collagen fibres in stress relaxation and stress distribution in the jaw-joint of rabbits. Arch Oral Biol. 1996;41:1039–52.
25. Tanaka E, Yamano E, Dalla-Bona DA, Watanabe M, Inubushi T, Shirakura M, et al. Dynamic compressive properties of the mandibular condylar cartilage. J Dent Res. 2006;85:571–5.
26. Tanaka E, van Eijden T. Biomechanical behavior of the temporomandibular joint disc. Crit Rev Oral Biol Med. 2003;14:138–50.
27. Sundblad L. Glycosaminoglycans and glycoproteins in synovial fluid. In: Balazs EA, Jeanloz RW, editors. The amino sugars. The chemistry and biology of compounds containing amino sugars. New York, NY: Academic Press; 1965. p. 229–50.
28. Yanaki T, Yamaguchi T. Temporary network formation of hyaluronate under a physiological condition. 1. Molecular-weight dependence. Biopolymers. 1990;30:415–25.
29. Kitamura R, Tanimoto K, Tanne Y, Kamiya T, Huang Y-C, Tanaka N, et al. Effects of mechanical load on the

expression and activity of hyaluronidase in cultured synovial membrane cells. J Biomed Mater Res. 2010;92A:87–93.

30. Itano N, Sawai T, Yoshida M, Lenas P, Yamada Y, Imagawa M, et al. Three isoforms of mammalian hyaluronan synthases have distinct enzymatic properties. J Biol Chem. 1999;274:25085–92.

31. Balazs E, Watson AD, Duff IF, Roseman S. Hyaluronic acid in synovial fluid. I. Molecular parameters of hyaluronic acid in normal and arthritis human fluids. Arthritis Rheum. 1967;10:357–76.

32. Yoshida M, Sai S, Marumo K, Tanaka T, Itano N, Kimata K, et al. Expression analysis of three isoforms of hyaluronan synthase and hyaluronidase in the synovium of knees in osteoarthritis and rheumatoid arthritis by quantitative real-time reverse transcriptase polymerase chain reaction. Arthritis Res Ther. 2004;6: R514–20.

33. Csoka AB, Frost GI, Stern R. The six hyaluronidase-like genes in the human and mouse genomes. Matrix Biol. 2001;20:499–508.

34. Nagaya H, Yamagata T, Yamagata S, Iyoda K, Ito H, Hasegawa Y, et al. Examination of synovial fluid and serum hyaluronidase activity as a joint marker in rheumatoid arthritis and osteoarthritis patients (by zymography). Ann Rheum Dis. 1999;58:186–8.

35. Carlsson GE, LeResche L. Epidemiology of temporomandibular disorders. In: Sessle BJ, Bryant PS, Dionne RA, editors. Temporomandibular disorders and related pain conditions. Seattle: Seattle Press; 1995.

36. Carlsson GE. Epidemiology and treatment need for temporomandibular disorders. J Orofac Pain. 1999;13:232–7.

37. Farrar WB, McCarty WL Jr. The TMJ dilemma. J Ala Dent Assoc. 1979;63:19–26.

38. Leonardi R, Lo Muzio L, Bernasconi G, Caltabiano C, Piacentini C, Caltabiano M. Expression of vascular endothelial growth factor in human dysfunctional temporomandibular joint disc. Arch Oral Biol. 2003;48:185–92.

39. Yoshida H, Fujita S, Nishida M, Iizuka T. Immunohistochemical distribution of lymph capillaries and blood capillaries in the synovial membrane in cases of internal derangement of the temporomandibular joint. J Oral Pathol Med. 1997;26:356–61.

40. Ghassemi-Nejad S, Kobezda T, Rauch TA, Matesz C, Grant TT, Mikecz K. Osteoarthritis-like damage of cartilage in the temporomandibular joints in mice with autoimmune inflammatory arthritis. Osteoarthr Cart. 2011;19:458–65.

41. Kubota E, Kubota T, Matsumoto J, Shibata T, Murakami K-I. Synovial fluid cytokines and proteinases as markers of temporomandibular joint disease. J Oral Maxillofac Surg. 1998;56:534–43.

42. Kuroda S, Tanimoto K, Izawa T, Fujihara S, Koolstra JH, Tanaka E. Biomechanical and biochemical characteristics of the mandibular condylar cartilage. Osteoarthr Cart. 2009;17:1408–15.

43. Kardel R, Ulfgren AK, Reinholt FP, Holmlund A. Inflammatory cell and cytokine patterns in patients with painful clicking and osteoarthritis in the temporomandibular joint. Int J Oral Maxillofac Surg. 2003;32:390–6.

44. Sato M, Nagata K, Kuroda S, Horiuchi S, Nakamura T, Karima M, et al. Low-intensity pulsed ultrasound activates integrin-mediated mechanotransduction pathway in synovial cells. Ann Biomed Eng. 2014;40:2156–63.

45. Scheven BA, Man J, Millard JL, Cooper PR, Lea SC, Walmsley AD, Smith AJ. VEGF and odontoblast-like cells: stimulation by low frequency ultrasound. Arch Oral Biol. 2009;54:185–91.

46. Neumann E, Lefèvre S, Zimmermann B, Gay S, Müller-Ladner U. Rheumatoid arthritis progression mediated by activated synovial fibroblasts. Trends Mol Med. 2010;16:458–68.

47. Scott DL, Wolfe F, Huizinga TW. Rheumatoid arthritis. Lancet. 2010;376:1094–108.

48. Audo R, Deschamps V, Hahne M, Combe B, Morel J. Apoptosis is not the major death mechanism induced by celecoxib on rheumatoid arthritis synovial fibroblasts. Arthritis Res Ther. 2007;9:R128.

49. Huber LC, Distler O, Tarner I, Gay RE, Gay S, Pap T. Synovial fibroblasts: key players in rheumatoid arthritis. Rheumatology. 2006;45:669–75.

50. Takeuchi R, Ryo A, Komitsu N, Mikuni-Takagaki Y, Fukui A, Takagi Y, et al. Low-intensity pulsed ultrasound activates the phosphatidylinositol 3 kinase/Akt pathway and stimulates the growth of chondrocytes in three-dimensional cultures: a basic science study. Arthritis Res Ther. 2008;10:R77.

51. Iwabuchi Y, Tanimoto K, Tanne Y, Inubushi T, Kamiya T, Huang YC, et al. Effects of low-intensity pulsed ultrasound on the expression of cyclooxygenase-2 in mandibular condylar chondrocytes. J Oral Facial Pain Headache. 2014;28:261–8.

52. El-Bialy TH, Elgazzar RF, Megahed EE, Royston TJ. Effects of ultrasound modes on mandibular osteodistraction. J Dent Res. 2008;87:953–7.

53. Huebner JL, Kraus VB. Assessment of the utility of biomarkers of osteoarthritis in the guinea pig. Osteoarthr Cart. 2006;14:923–30.

54. Konttinen YT, Saari H, Nordstrom DC. Effect of interleukin-1 on hyaluronate synthesis by synovial fibroblastic cells. Clin Rheumatol. 1991;10:151–4.

55. Sampson PM, Rochester CL, Freundlich B, Elias JA. Cytokine regulation of human lung fibroblast hyaluronan (hyaluronic acid) production. Evidence for cytokine-regulated hyaluronan (hyaluronic acid) degradation and human lung fibroblast-derived hyaluronidase. J Clin Invest. 1992;90:1492–503.

56. Nakamura T, Fujihara S, Katsura T, Yamamoto K, Inubushi T, Tanimoto K, Tanaka E. Effects of low-intensity pulsed ultrasound on the expression and activity of hyaluronic synthase and hyaluronidase in

IL-1β-stimulated synovial cells. Ann Biomed Eng. 2010;38:3363–70.

57. Lal H, Verma SK, Smith M, Guleria RS, Lu G, Foster DM, Dostal DE. Stretch-induced MAP kinase activation in cardiac myocytes: differential regulation through beta 1-integrin and focal adhesion kinase. J Mol Cell Cardiol. 2007;43:137–47.

58. Zhou S, Schmelz A, Seufferlein T, Li Y, Zhao J, Bachem MG. Molecular mechanisms of low intensity pulsed ultrasound in human skin fibroblasts. J Biol Chem. 2004;279:54463–9.

59. Hsu HC, Fong YC, Chang CS, Hsu CJ, Hsu SF, Lin JG, et al. Ultrasound induces cyclooxygenase-2-expression through integrin, integrin-linked kinase, Akt, NF-κB and p300 pathway in human chondrocytes. Cell Signal. 2007;19:2317–28.

60. Rego EB, Inubushi T, Kawazoe A, Tanimoto K, Miyauchi M, Tanaka E, et al. Ultrasound stimulation induces PGE_2 synthesis promoting cementoblastic differentiation through EP2/EP4 receptor pathway. Ultrasound Med Biol. 2010;36:907–15.

61. El-Bialy T, El-Shamy I, Graber TM. Growth modification of the rabbit mandible using therapeutic ultrasound: is it possible to enhance functional appliance results? Angle Orthod. 2003;73:631–9.

62. Oyonarte R, Zárate M, Rodriguez F. Low-intensity pulsed ultrasound stimulation of condylar growth in rats. Angle Orthod. 2009;79:964–70.

63. Oyonarte R, Becerra D, Díaz-Zúñiga J, Rojas V, Carrion F. Morphological effects of mesenchymal stem cells and pulsed ultrasound on condylar growth in rats: a pilot study. Aust Orthod J. 2013;29:3–12.

64. Chan CW, Qin L, Lee KM, Cheung WH, Cheng JCY, Leung KS. Dose-dependent effect of low-intensity pulsed ultrasound on callus formation during rapid distraction osteogenesis. J Orthop Res. 2006;24:2072–9.

65. El-Bialy TH, Royston TJ, Magin RL, Evans CA, Zaki A-M, Frizzell LA. The effect of pulsed ultrasound on mandibular distraction. Ann Biomed Eng. 2002;30:1251–61.

66. Schumann D, Kujat R, Zellner J, Angele MK, Nerlich M, Mayr E, et al. Treatment of human mesenchymal stem cells with pulsed low intensity ultrasound enhances the chondrogenic phenotype in vitro. Biorheology. 2006;43:431–43.

67. Kaur H, Uludağ H, Dederich DN, El-Bialy T. Effect of increasing low-intensity pulsed ultrasound and a functional appliance on the mandibular condyle in growing rats. J Ultrasound Med. 2017;36:109–20.

68. Kaur H, Uludağ H, El-Bialy T. Effect of nonviral plasmid delivered basic fibroblast growth factor and low intensity pulsed ultrasound on mandibular condylar growth: a preliminary study. Biomed Res Int. 2014;2014:426710.

69. Nakamura T, Fujihara S, Yamamoto-Nagata K, Katsura T, Inubushi T, Tanaka E. Low-intensity pulsed ultrasound reduces the inflammatory activity of synovitis. Ann Biomed Eng. 2011;39:2964–71.

Application of LIPUS to Salivary Glands

Minami Sato, Toshihiro Inubushi, and Eiji Tanaka

Abstract

Sjögren syndrome (SS) is one of the most common unexplained intractable autoimmune diseases occurring in middle-aged women. Patients with SS manifest progressive dryness symptoms due to insufficient salivary and lacrimal secretions. Xerostomia, defined as dry mouth, is a subjective symptom that most commonly appears in SS patients. Available causal treatment of xerostomia has been limited, and then the establishment of a causal treatment with no or less side effect is urgently needed. The effect of noninvasive low-intensity pulsed ultrasound (LIPUS) on soft tissues has received much attention for promoting effects on soft tissue healing. Thus, LIPUS may have considerable clinical potential for treatment of injured or pathological soft tissues including salivary gland. Recently, we investigated the effects of LIPUS on salivary gland cells and demonstrated that the expression of aquaporin 5 (AQP5), a water channel protein, in human salivary gland acinar cells was inhibited by TNF-α treatment, whereas it was recovered following LIPUS treatment. In addition, our in vivo study using MRL/*lpr* mice, the best model for SS, suggests that LIPUS treatment restored salivary gland secretion volumes in older MRL/*lpr* mice, thereby promoting an anti-inflammatory response and improving AQP5 dysfunction. It is concluded that LIPUS stimulation may represent a treatment strategy for inflammatory diseases of salivary glands, including xerostomia in SS.

M. Sato
Department of Orthodontics and Dentofacial Orthopedics, Institute of Biomedical Sciences, Tokushima University Graduate School, Tokushima, Japan

T. Inubushi
Genetic Disease Program, Sanford Children's Health Research Center, Sanford-Burnham Medical Research Institute, La Jolla, CA, USA

E. Tanaka (✉)
Department of Orthodontics and Dentofacial Orthopedics, Institute of Biomedical Sciences, Tokushima University Graduate School, Tokushima, Japan

Department of Orthodontics, King Abdulaziz University, Jeddah, Saudi Arabia
e-mail: etanaka@tokushima-u.ac.jp

7.1 Introduction

Salivary glands are complex exocrine glands consisting of three major salivary glands: parotid gland, submandibular gland and sublingual gland, and other small salivary glands (Fig. 7.1). Salivary glands secrete saliva composed of at least 99% water. Sjögren syndrome (SS) is one of the most common unexplained intractable autoimmune diseases occurring in middle-aged women and characterized by lymphocytic infiltrates and destruction of salivary and lacrimal glands

© Springer International Publishing AG, part of Springer Nature 2018
T. El-Bialy et al. (eds.), *Therapeutic Ultrasound in Dentistry*,
https://doi.org/10.1007/978-3-319-66323-4_7

Fig. 7.1 Anatomy of the salivary glands. The major salivary glands include parotid gland, sublingual gland, and submandibular gland

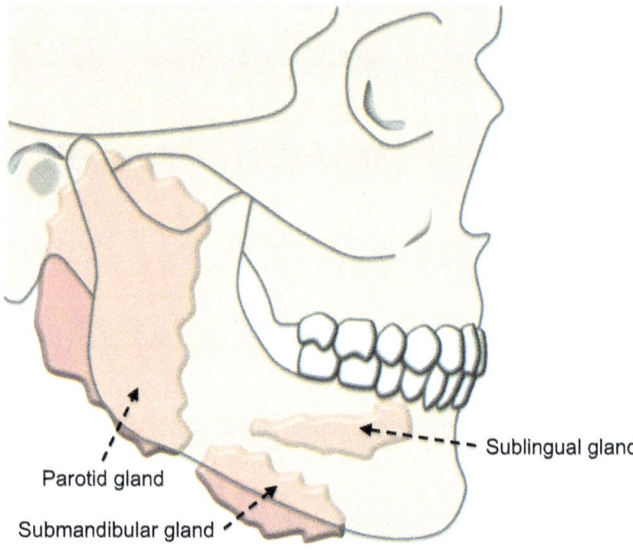

Fig. 7.2 The common symptoms of SS. Dry mouth most frequently appears as a subjective symptom of SS and seriously decreases patient's QOL by various symptoms

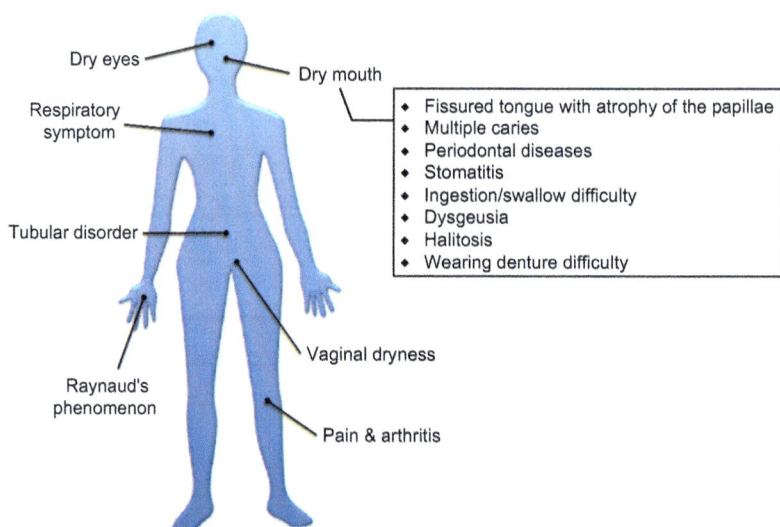

[1, 2]. Patients with SS manifest progressive dryness symptoms due to insufficient salivary and lacrimal secretions [3]: dry mouth, dry eyes, respiratory symptom, Raynaud's phenomenon, tubular disorder, vagital dryness, arthritis, and more (Fig. 7.2). Among them, dry mouth is a subjective symptom that most commonly appears in SS patients.

Xerostomia is defined as dry mouth resulting from reduced or absent salivary flow. It induces various symptoms: fissured tongue with atrophy of the papillae, multiple caries, periodontal diseases, stomatitis, ingestion/swallow difficulty, dysgeusia, halitosis, and difficulty in wearing dentures. As a result, patient's "quality of life (QOL)" is seriously decreased.

Currently, the cause of xerostomia experienced by patients with SS remains unknown. However, dynamic expression of various cytokines has been detected in the salivary glands of humans, as well as in experimental animals, during the development of SS [4, 5]. In particular, expression of tumor necrosis factor-α (TNF-α) has been strongly associated with decreased salivary flow in patients with SS [6]. It is indicated that TNF-α inhibits salivary secretion due to its neurotoxic effect on sympathetic nerves. Aquaporin 5 (AQP5), a water channel protein, facilitates the rapid transcellular movement of water in response to osmotic and/or hydrostatic pressure gradients [7]. On the basis of its reduced expression and abnormal distribution in the salivary and lacrimal glands of patients with SS, a potential role of AQP5 is proposed.

Available treatment of xerostomia is divided into two types: symptomatic and causal treatments. The former treatment includes artificial saliva, troche, oral ointment, and gargle. However, the purpose of these treatments is only to moisten the oral cavity and not to improve the salivary secretion. The latter includes salivator and herbal medicine. Hydroxychloroquine (HCQ), one of the most frequently proposed treatments for SS, is currently used on the basis of data obtained from an observational study [8] and a crossover study [9]. However, in a more recent randomized controlled study, the primary endpoint was not achieved [10]. In a recent clinical report regarding the chimeric anti-TNF-α antibody infliximab, patients with SS were found to exhibit a dramatic improvement in salivary flow [11], though there have been few scattered reports of anti-TNF-α treatment inefficacy [12, 13]. Furthermore, Yamamura et al. [3] found that TNF-α stimulation dramatically decreased water flow rate (e.g., salivary flow) in cultured acinar cells of human salivary glands, supporting the effectiveness of infliximab. Thus, accumulating evidence suggests that anti-cytokine therapy including targeted inhibition of TNF-α activity may represent a treatment for xerostomia caused by autoimmune sialadenitis in SS. However, anti-TNF-α treatment has multiple potential adverse effects, including anaphylaxis [14], and increased risk for infections, such as tuberculosis and demyelination, aplastic anemia, intestinal perforation, lymphoma, and congestive heart failure [15]. Taken together, the establishment of a treatment with no or less side effect is urgently needed.

Recently, the effect of noninvasive low-intensity pulsed ultrasound (LIPUS) on soft tissues has received much attention for promoting effects on soft tissue healing. Furthermore, it has been shown that LIPUS reduces inflammation and promotes regeneration in various injured soft tissues [16–20]. Thus, LIPUS may have considerable clinical potential for treatment of injured or pathological soft tissues including salivary gland.

Lately, we have investigated the effects of LIPUS on salivary gland cells and examined the therapeutic effects [21]. In the study, human salivary gland acinar (NS-SV-AC) cells were cultured with or without 10 ng/ml TNF-α followed by a single LIPUS exposure or sham exposure. In addition, we analyzed the effect of LIPUS on the nuclear factor κB (NF-κB) signaling pathway in NS-SV-AC cells stimulated with TNF-α. Moreover, the effectiveness of LIPUS in recovering salivary secretion was examined in an MRL/MpJ/*lpr/lpr* (MRL/*lpr*) mouse model of SS with autoimmune sialadenitis.

7.2 Effects of LIPUS on Salivary Gland Cells

We first examined the effects of LIPUS on proliferation of NS-SV-AC cells by WST-8 assay (Fig. 7.3a). Compared with the untreated control, stimulation with TNF-α resulted in a significant decrease in cell proliferation of NS-SV-AC cells, but LIPUS significantly ($p < 0.05$) upregulated the proliferation of NS-SV-AC cells stimulated with TNF-α. Furthermore, the subsequent LIPUS treatment induced a significant increase in proliferation for NS-SV-AC cells stimulated with TNF-α ($p < 0.01$). Treatment with LIPUS alone had no catabolic effect on cell proliferation.

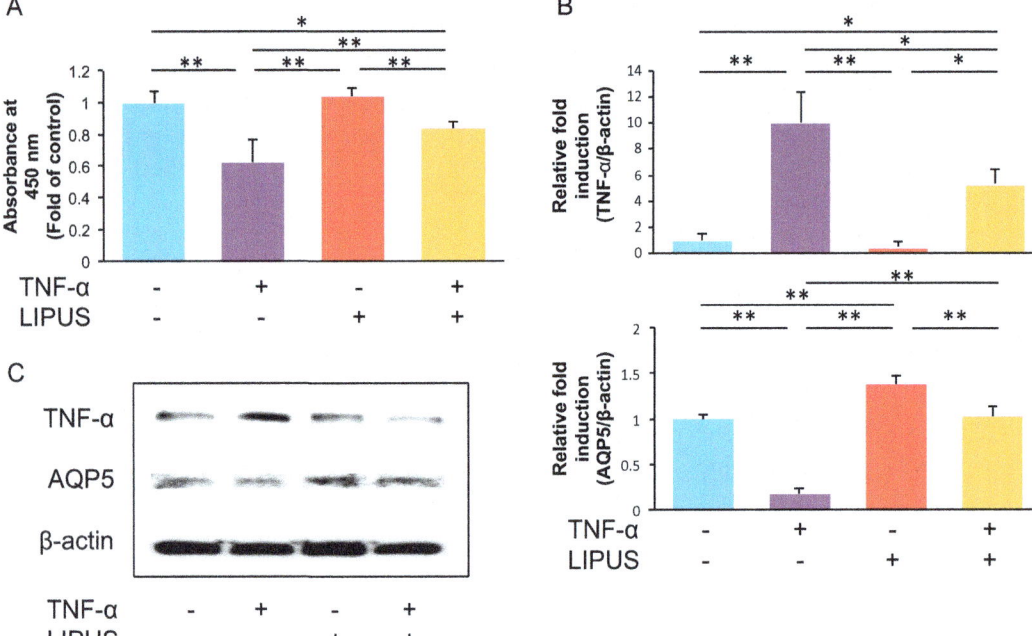

Fig. 7.3 Effects of LIPUS on NS-SV-AC cells. (**a**) WST-8 assay showing a significant decrease in cell proliferation by TNF-α stimulation and increased following LIPUS treatment. (**b**) TNF-α stimulation of NS-SV-AC cells significantly increased levels of *TNF-α* mRNA and decreased levels of *AQP5* mRNA. Detection of *β-actin* mRNA was used to calculate relative fold induction for each. However, when TNF-α stimulation was followed by LIPUS, both levels were restored to those of control cells. (**c**) In Western blot assays, the expression of the AQP5 was decreased following TNF-α stimulation, whereas the expression of TNF-α was increased. When LIPUS was performed following TNF-α treatment, levels of AQP5 were increased compared with untreated controls. *$p < 0.05$; **$p < 0.01$ as tested with Tukey–Kramer and Bonferroni/Dunn test ($n = 6$). (Modified from Sato et al. [21])

We next investigated the effect of LIPUS on the expression of AQP5, a marker for salivary secretion, and TNF-α in NS-SV-AC cells by real-time PCR and Western blot analysis. Compared with control cells, the stimulation of NS-SV-AC cells with TNF-α resulted in a significant decrease in expression level of *AQP5* mRNA ($p < 0.01$) and a significant increase in expression level of *TNF-α* mRNA ($p < 0.01$) (Fig. 7.3b). However, the latter was reversed following treatment with LIPUS ($p < 0.05$). In Western blot analysis, the intensity of the AQP5 band detected was decreased following TNF-α stimulation, whereas expression of TNF-α was clearly enhanced (Fig. 7.3c). However, when LIPUS was exposed to the cells treated with TNF-α, an increase in AQP5 level was observed in NS-SV-AC cells extracts compared with untreated control cells. In contrast, AQP5 levels of untreated cells that received LIPUS treatment alone exhibited minimal, if any, change in signal intensity.

These data show that the expression of AQP5 in NS-SV-AC cells was inhibited by TNF-α treatment, whereas it was recovered following LIPUS treatment.

7.3 Mechanism of LIPUS on Salivary Gland Cell's Function

We speculated that the result of in vitro study is due to the anti-inflammatory effects of LIPUS treatment on the inflamed salivary gland cells via the prevention of NF-κB activation.

NF-κB is composed of homo- and heterodimeric complexes of members of the Rel protein family. NF-κB normally resides in the cytoplasm, where it is inactivated by IκB protein, an endogenous inhibitor. Various extracellular stimuli trigger the degradation of IκB by the proteasome pathway. Subsequently, NF-κB released from IκB translocates into the nucleus, binds to the regulatory element of the target genes, and controls their transcription [22] (Fig. 7.4a).

Accordingly, we investigated the anti-inflammatory effect of LIPUS on the phosphorylation of IκBα, NF-κB, and IKKβ (Fig. 7.4b). Western blot analysis showed that IκBα, NF-κB, and IKKβ phosphorylation was obviously induced by TNF-α stimulation; however, LIPUS treatment inhibited IκBα, NF-κB, and IKKβ phosphorylation. In addition, IκBα, NF-κB, and IKKβ phosphorylation induced by IL-1β stimulation was also inhibited by LIPUS treatment. This indicates that anti-inflammatory effects of LIPUS are not a specific response to TNF-α stimulation. A20 is known as the intracellular ubiquitin-editing protein and a key player in the negative feedback of NF-κB signaling in response to multiple stimulations [23]. Therefore, we examined A20 (tumor necrosis factor-α-induced protein 3 [TNFAIP3]) mRNA expression using a real-time PCR. Compared with untreated control cells, the stimulation of NS-SV-AC cells with TNF-α or IL-1β resulted in a significant increase in expression level of A20 mRNA (Fig. 7.4c). However, A20 mRNA expression was significantly higher in LIPUS-treated groups. These data show that LIPUS enhances production of A20, the negative feedback regulator of NF-κB signaling, resulting in inhibition of inflammation in salivary gland cells.

7.4 In Vivo Study

One of the best models for SS is MRL/*lpr* mice, since marked infiltration of lymphocytes has been reported in lacrimal and salivary glands, and it resembles human SS. To examine the effect of LIPUS on salivary gland inflammation, lacrimal gland dysfunction manifested by xerostomia in MRL/*lpr* mice, secreted saliva volumes were measured using a modified method employed in the Saxon test [24, 25]. MRL/*lpr* mice exhibited a significant increase in salivary secretion following LIPUS treatment compared with untreated MRL/*lpr* mice (Fig. 7.5a). The salivary glands in MRL/*lpr* mice treated with LIPUS showed a marked reduction in histological damage, such as the lymphocyte infiltration of surrounding duct and the destruction of gland tissue, compared with untreated MRL/*lpr* mice. Moreover, histological grading was performed according to a previously proposed method [26]. The histological score for the inflammatory lesions of the submandibular glands of MRL/*lpr* mice was significantly improved by the LIPUS treatment ($p < 0.05$) (Fig. 7.5b).

Following LIPUS treatment, significantly lower level of TNF-α ($p < 0.05$) and significantly higher level of AQP5 ($p < 0.05$) were detected in the salivary glands (Fig. 7.5c). As shown in Fig. 7.5d, submandibular gland acinar cells of untreated MRL/*lpr* mice showed weak staining for AQP5 expression (brown stain) in the submandibular glands. In contrast, strong expression of AQP5 was observed at apical sites in submandibular gland acinar cells of MRL/*lpr* mice treated with LIPUS. These results suggest that LIPUS might rescue salivary secretion volume in an SS mouse model via their anti-inflammatory effect in the salivary gland tissue.

7.5 Clinical Application of LIPUS to Xerostomia in SS Patients

The drug therapy of SS patients still remains challenging because the common side effect of many drugs is dryness of the mucous membrane. It is also notable that SS patients are more susceptible to drug allergies. However, the establishment of an effective treatment with low side effect is strongly desired to improve QOL in SS patients.

LIPUS is a method of treating specific area of the body with daily short-time, usually 20 min, application of pulsed ultrasound. It is also a great advantage that only a simple instrument is required to operate and install. In addition, LIPUS is possible to use in combination with

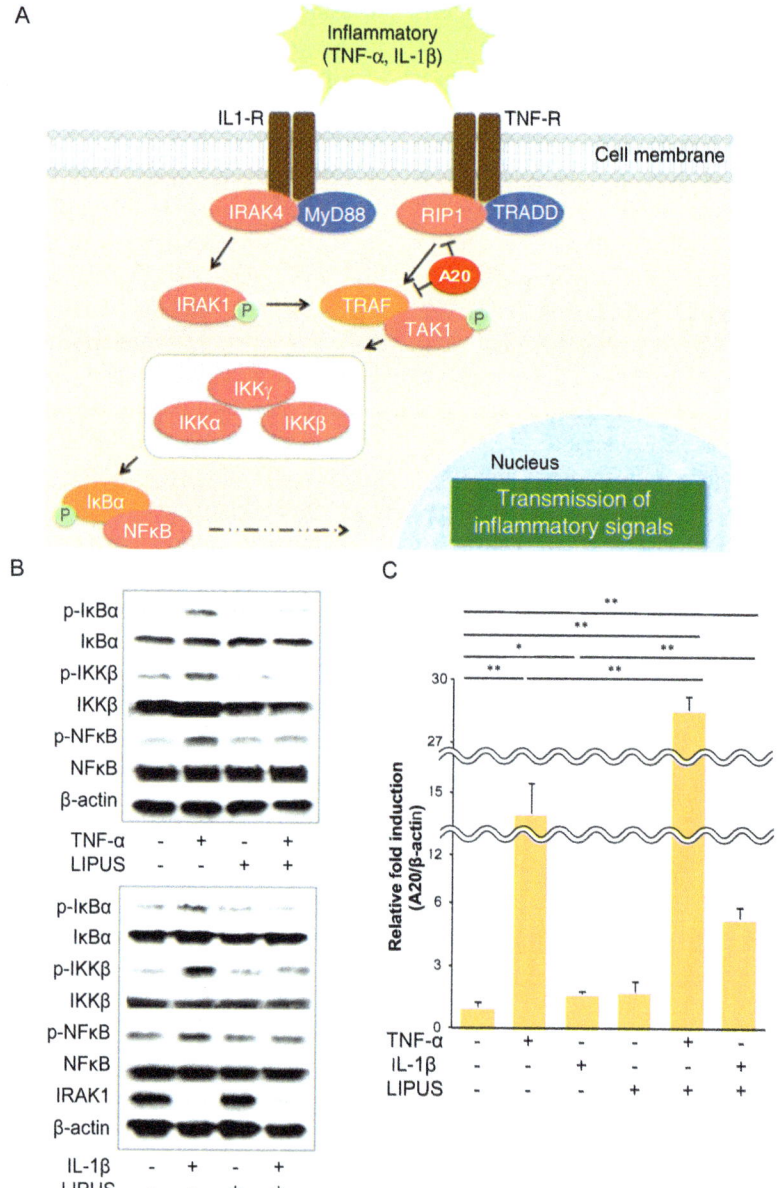

Fig. 7.4 Anti-inflammatory mechanism of LIPUS on NS-SV-AC cellular function. (a) Schematic illustration of anti-inflammatory mechanisms of NF-κB pathways. (b) Western blot analysis showing that IκBα phosphorylation was obviously induced by TNF-α stimulation; however, when LIPUS treatment was administered following TNF-α treatment, IκBα, NF-κB, and IKKβ phosphorylation were inhibited. Similar inhibitory effects of LIPUS were observed in IL-1β stimulation. Moreover, IRAK1 was degraded after IL-1β stimulation, and LIPUS treatment failed to inhibit it. (c) The stimulation of NS-SV-AC cells with TNF-α or IL-1β resulted in a significant increase in levels of *A20* mRNA, and *A20* mRNA expression was further increased following treatment with LIPUS after TNF-α or IL-1β stimulation. *$p < 0.05$; **$p < 0.01$ as tested with Tukey–Kramer and Bonferroni/Dunn test ($n = 6$). (Modified from Sato et al. [21])

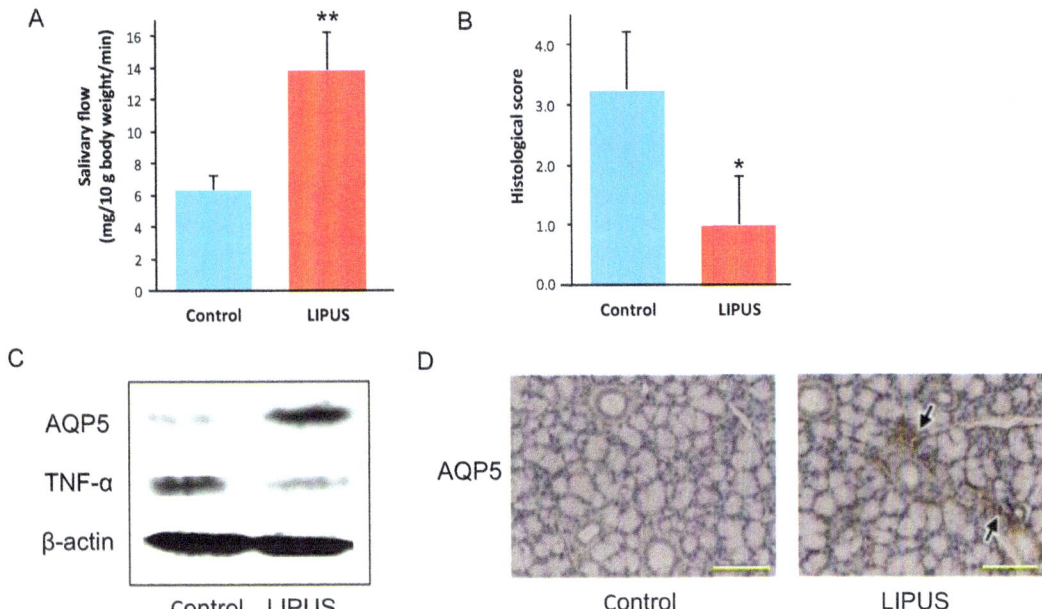

Fig. 7.5 In vivo effects of LIPUS on MRL/*lpr* mice. (**a**) MRL/*lpr* mice showed a significant increase in salivary flow following LIPUS treatment. (**b**) Histological scores for inflammatory lesions present in the salivary glands of untreated versus LIPUS-treated MRL/*lpr* mice. LIPUS treatment significantly improved the histological score. *$p < 0.05$; **$p < 0.01$ as tested with Tukey–Kramer and Bonferroni/Dunn test ($n = 5$). (**c**) In Western blot assays, levels of TNF-α were lower and AQP5 were higher following LIPUS treatment compared with untreated MRL/*lpr* samples. Detection of β-actin was used to calculate relative fold induction for each. (**d**) In the submandibular glands, acinar cells of untreated MRL/*lpr* mice exhibited weak staining for AQP5, whereas intense staining of AQP5 was localized to apical sites in acinar cells of MRL/*lpr* mice treated with LIPUS (arrows). Scale bar = 100 μm. (Modified from Sato et al. [21])

conventional drug therapy. Therefore, we believe that introduction of LIPUS can reduce the dose of drug having adverse effects and shorten the period until the effect appears. In addition, LIPUS is a simple instrument to operate and install. We expect that clinical application of LIPUS can be glad tidings.

Recently, we have started clinical trial on the effectiveness of the combination of cepharanthin, promising drug to improve salivary secretion in SS patients [27], and LIPUS for SS patients. We would like to establish the clinical application of LIPUS by examining experimental conditions.

7.6 Conclusions

LIPUS treatment was found to increase cell proliferation and AQP5 expression in salivary gland cells pretreated with TNF-α in vitro. Moreover, LIPUS activates the intracellular ubiquitin-editing protein A20, which produces negative feedback of NF-κB signaling in response to inflammatory stimulation. LIPUS treatment also restored salivary gland secretion volumes in older MRL/*lpr* mice in vivo, thereby promoting an anti-inflammatory response and improving AQP5 dysfunction. Therefore, LIPUS stimulation may represent a treatment strategy for inflammatory diseases of salivary glands, including xerostomia in SS.

References

1. Fox RI. Sjögren's syndrome. Lancet. 2005;366:321–31.
2. Daniels TE. Labial salivary gland biopsy in Sjögren's syndrome: assessment as a diagnostic criterion in 362 suspected cases. Arthritis Rheum. 1984;27:147–56.
3. Yamamura Y, Motegi K, Kani K, Takano H, Momota Y, Aota K, et al. TNF-α inhibits aquaporin 5 expression in human salivary gland acinar cells via

suppression of histone H4 acetylation. J Cell Mol Med. 2012;16:1766–75.

4. Fox RI, Kang HI, Ando D, Abrams J, Pisa E. Cytokine mRNA expression in salivary gland biopsies of Sjögren's syndrome. J Immunol. 1994;152:5532–9.

5. Hamano H, Saito I, Haneji N, Mitsuhashi Y, Miyasaka N, Hayashi Y. Expressions of cytokine genes during development of autoimmune sialadenitis in MRL/lpr mice. Eur J Immunol. 1993;23:2387–91.

6. Soliven B, Wang N. Tumor necrosis factor-α regulates nicotinic responses in mixed cultures of sympathetic neurons and nonneuronal cells. J Neurochem. 1995;64:883–94.

7. King LS, Yasui M. Aquaporins and disease: lessons from mice to humans. Trends Endocrinol Metab. 2002;13:355–60.

8. Fox RI, Dixon R, Guarrasi V, Krubel S. Treatment of primary Sjögren's syndrome with hydroxychloroquine: a retrospective, open-label study. Lupus. 1996;5 (Suppl 1):S31–6.

9. Kruize AA, Hené RJ, Kallenberg CG, van Bijsterveld OP, van der Heide A, Kater L, et al. Hydroxychloroquine treatment for primary Sjögren's syndrome: a two year double blind crossover trial. Ann Rheum Dis. 1993;52:360–4.

10. Gottenberg JE, Ravaud P, Puéchal X, Le Guern V, Sibilia J, Goeb V, et al. Effects of hydroxychloroquine on symptomatic improvement in primary Sjögren syndrome: the JOQUER randomized clinical trial. JAMA. 2014;312:249–58.

11. Steinfeld SD, Demols P, Salmon I, Kiss R, Appelboom T. Infliximab in patients with primary Sjögren's syndrome: a pilot study. Arthritis Rheum. 2001;44:2371–5.

12. Mariette X, Ravaud P, Steinfeld S, Baron G, Goetz J, Hachulla E, et al. Inefficacy of infliximab in primary Sjögren's syndrome: results of the randomized, controlled Trial of Remicade in Primary Sjögren's Syndrome (TRIPSS). Arthritis Rheum. 2004;50:1270–6.

13. Sankar V, Brennan MT, Kok MR, Leakan RA, Smith JA, Manny J, et al. Etanercept in Sjögren's syndrome: a twelve-week randomized, double-blind, placebo-controlled pilot clinical trial. Arthritis Rheum. 2004;50:2240–5.

14. Desai D, Goldbach-Mansky R, Milner JD, Rabin RL, Hull K, Pucino F, et al. Anaphylactic reaction to anakinra in a rheumatoid arthritis patient intolerant to multiple nonbiologic and biologic disease-modifying antirheumatic drugs. Ann Pharmacother. 2009;43:967–72.

15. Antoni C, Braun J. Side effects of anti TNF therapy: current knowledge. Clin Exp Rheumatol. 2002;20: S152–7.

16. Nagata K, Nakamura T, Fujihara S, Tanaka E. Ultrasound modulates the inflammatory response and promotes muscle regeneration in injured muscles. Ann Biomed Eng. 2013;41:1095–105.

17. Nakamura T, Fujihara S, Katsura T, Yamamoto K, Inubushi T, Tanimoto K, et al. Effects of low-intensity pulsed ultrasound on the expression and activity of hyaluronan synthase and hyaluronidase in IL-1β-stimulated synovial cells. Ann Biomed Eng. 2010;38:3363–70.

18. Nakamura T, Fujihara S, Yamamoto-Nagata K, Katsura T, Inubushi T, Tanaka E. Low-intensity pulsed ultrasound reduces the inflammatory activity of synovitis. Ann Biomed Eng. 2011;39:2964–71.

19. Tanaka E, Kuroda S, Horiuchi S, Tabata A, El-Bialy T. Low-intensity pulsed ultrasound in dentofacial tissue engineering. Ann Biomed Eng. 2015;43:871–86.

20. Takakura Y, Matsui N, Yoshiya S, Fujioka H, Muratsu H, Tsunoda M, et al. Low-intensity pulsed ultrasound enhances early healing of medial collateral ligament injuries in rats. J Ultrasound Med. 2002;21:283–8.

21. Sato M, Kuroda S, Mansjur KQ, Ganzorig K, Nagata K, Horiuchi S, et al. Low-intensity pulsed ultrasound rescues insufficient salivary secretion in autoimmune sialadenitis. Arthritis Res Ther. 2015;17:278.

22. Barnes PJ, Karin M. Nuclear factor-κB: a pivotal transcription factor in chronic inflammatory diseases. N Engl J Med. 1997;336:1066–71.

23. Vereecke L, Beyaert R, van Loo G. The ubiquitin-editing enzyme A20 (TNFAIP3) is a central regulator of immunopathology. Trends Immunol. 2009;30:383–91.

24. Delporte C, O'Connell BC, He X, Lancaster HE, O'Connell AC, Agre P, et al. Increased fluid secretion after adenoviral-mediated transfer of the aquaporin-1 cDNA to irradiated rat salivary glands. Proc Natl Acad Sci USA. 1997;94:3268–73.

25. Kohler PF, Winter ME. A quantitative test for xerostomia: the Saxon test, an oral equivalent of the Schirmer test. Arthritis Rheum. 1985;28:1128–32.

26. White SC, Casarett GW. Damage of rat thyroid by ^{131}I and evidence against immunologic transferability. Radiat Res. 1974;57:288–99.

27. Yamanoi T, Aota K, Momota Y, Azuma M. Treatment with the biscoclaurine alkaloid Cepharanthin Significantly Increases Salivary Secretion in Primary Sjögren's Syndrome Patients. J Oral Health Biosci. 2017;29:39–48.

Application of LIPUS in Orthodontics

8

Tarek El-Bialy

Abstract

Since 2002, when the first scientific paper on the effect of LIPUS on lower incisors eruption and formation was reported, an extensive research has been conducted to understand the mechanism by which LIPUS can stimulate dental forming cells to produce dental tissues, in particular dentine and cementum. Also, it was back in 1971 when it was reported that ultrasound can alter growing end plates in small animals, the concept that can be and has been utilized in the lower arch to modify its growth at both the experimental and clinical trials levels. This chapter will shed light on the current evidence in the literature that suggests the use of LIPUS in daily orthodontic practices in many applications.

8.1 Introduction

Orthodontics is the art and science that deals with correcting crowded teeth, abnormal teeth bites, and jaw mal-relationships. Orthodontics involve harmonizing teeth position, jaw position, and circumoral muscles and takes into consideration jaw position/changes (jaw orthopedics) in growing children or in adults that may involve adjunctive surgical procedures. Orthodontics also involves management and correction of abnormal teeth positions and malocclusion. Dental malocclusion can be due to congenital or environmental factors. Correcting abnormal teeth position involves application of mechanical forces that are intended to change teeth and/or jaw positions using fixed or removable orthodontic/orthopedic appliances that are intended to move the teeth or change positions of the jaws. The mechanical forces are applied to induce biomechanical stimuli in the bone, and hence tooth movement occurs. Some malocclusions are hard to be corrected solely by orthodontic appliances especially in cases with small size jaws or when the jaws are positioned far from each other. In these cases, orthopedic appliances may modify the position of the jaw while the patients are still growing, while in adults jaw position is best corrected by surgical intervention. This chapter will shed light on challenges in orthodontics and how low-intensity pulsed ultrasound may provide solutions in some cases where challenges are encountered.

8.1.1 Orthodontic Tooth Movement

Orthodontic tooth movement is considered as a sterile induced inflammatory process to induce biochemical reaction to the applied orthodontic

T. El-Bialy (✉)
Dentistry/Orthodontics and Biomedical Engineering, University of Alberta, Edmonton, Alberta, Canada
e-mail: telbialy@ualberta.ca

© Springer International Publishing AG, part of Springer Nature 2018
T. El-Bialy et al. (eds.), *Therapeutic Ultrasound in Dentistry*,
https://doi.org/10.1007/978-3-319-66323-4_8

forces. These reactions are the basis of inducing stimulating differentiation of bone formation and bone resorption at the same time; hence, teeth move within the remodeled alveolar bone/periodontal ligament. During orthodontic tooth movement, the inflammatory processes induced by orthodontic forces that are responsible for differentiating the mesenchymal cells into osteoblasts and recruitment of osteoclasts at the same factors that have been reported to be involved in cementoclasts and/or odontoclasts. These cells are involved in tooth root resorption.

8.1.2 Orthodontically Induced Inflammatory Root Resorption

OIIRR is the second most common unavoidable side effect of orthodontic tooth movement. The frequency of incisors having root resorption has been shown to be increased from 15% before treatment to 73% after treatment [1] and in another study from none before treatment to more than 80% after treatment [2]. This relationship includes the severity as well as the extension, where the number of teeth with moderate and severe root resorption increased from 1% before treatment to 25% after treatment [1]. In addition, it has been reported that about 4% of orthodontic patients show generalized resorption of the six anterior teeth of more than 3 mm [3]. Other studies have shown that about 5% of adults [4] and only 2% of adolescents [5] are likely to have at least one tooth that shows severe resorption more than 5 mm during treatment. The incidences of severe root resorption have been reported to be more frequent in the apical one-third of the involved teeth [6].

Although there are many hypotheses about the etiologic factors that might contribute to the occurrence of severe OIIRR, there is no clear cause and effect relationship between the possible etiologic factors and severe OIIRR. Osteoclastogenesis was reported to be related to the balance between receptor activator of nuclear factor kappa B (NF-κB) ligand (RANKL) and osteoprotegerin (OPG) expression in osteoblasts, where OPG decreases osteoclastogenesis and RANKL

increases it [7, 8]. Furthermore, it has been reported that OPG/RANK/RANKL pathway that controls the osteoclastogenesis and odontoclastogenesis has been reported to exist in physiologic root resorption in deciduous teeth [9]. RANKL and OPG levels have been reported to increase during the application of heavy forces and severe root resorption [10–13]. In addition, PDL cells obtained from patients with severe OIIRR showed increased production of RANKL and low expression of OPG, which stimulated osteoclast formation [13].

Management of OIIRR include allowing for self-healing for 70 days [14], or after retention [15]; application of bisphosphonate to rats' teeth [16]; topical corticosteroid ([17]; root canal treatment with calcium hydroxide [18]; and recently low-intensity pulsed ultrasound (LIPUS) in humans ([19, 20], [Fig. 8.1]) and in experimental animals ([21–24], [Fig. 8.2]). Although the exact mechanism by which LIPUS minimizes OIIRR is not fully understood, it has been reported that the effect of LIPUS in minimizing OIIRR is multifactorial. Studies have shown that LIPUS modulates the OPG/RANK/RANKL balance and hence minimizes osteoclastogenesis, as well as LIPUS has been shown to increase cementum formation and predentine/dentine in experimental animals and in humans [19, 23–27]. Detailed review of LIPUS effect on prevention/minimizing OIRR has been presented in Chap. 7. This evidence has been supported by other study that showed that LIPUS enhanced cementoblasts differentiation [28].

Accelerated tooth movement during orthodontic treatment has received a great deal of attention recently with the aim to minimize possible OIRR, loss of patient compliance, and other side effects of prolonged orthodontic treatment like enamel decalcification, periodontitis, and patient psychological impact. The current reported data about techniques that can accelerate tooth movement include microosteoperforation, high frequency vibration (Vpro5, Propel Inc., USA), photobiomodulation (Orthopulse, Biolux) and low intensity pulsed ultrasound [LIPUS] (AEVO system, SmileSonica Inc., Edmonton, Alberta, Canada).

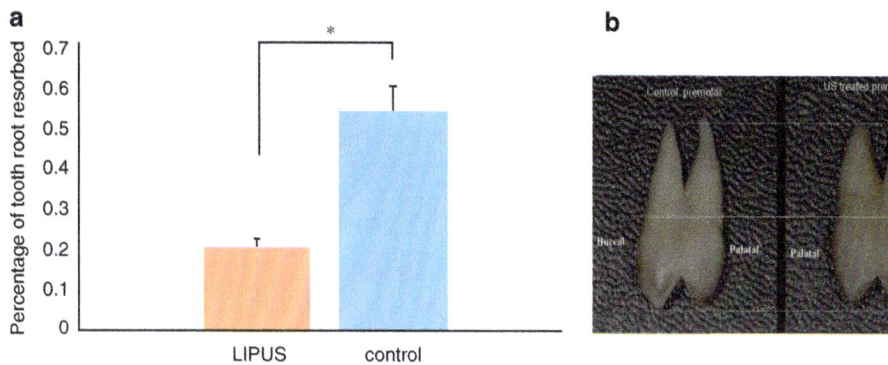

Fig. 8.1 (**a**) Total volume of RL (mm3) (mean +/− SE) in LIPUS and control group (*$p < 0.05$) (From [20]). (**b**) An example of LIPUS-treated and control premolars. It can be seen that LIPUS-treated premolar (right) did not show severe root resorption like the control premolar (left)

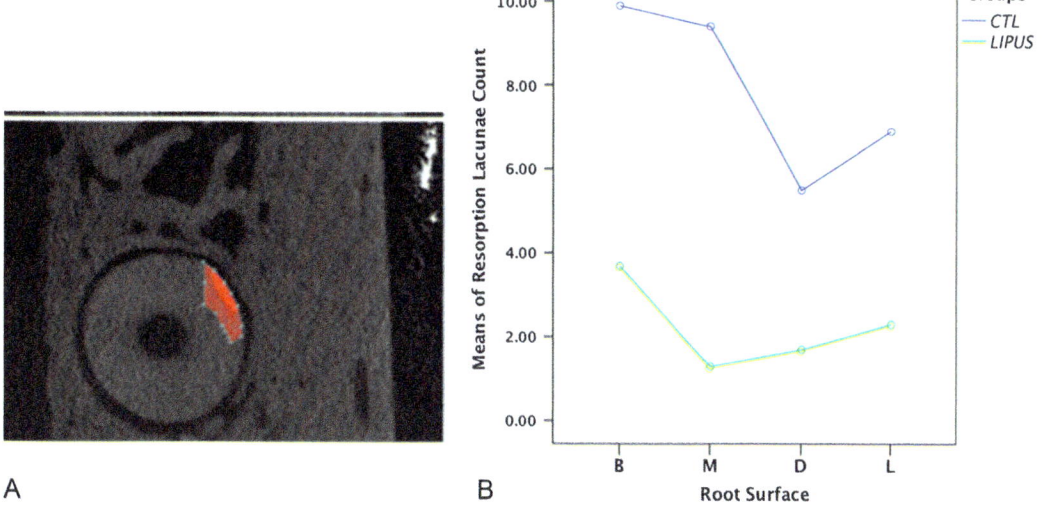

Fig. 8.2 (**a**) Cross-sectional view of the beagle dog root with the highlighted region of interest covering the resorption lacunae for volumetric measurements. (**b**) Comparison of OIRR between LIPUS-treated and control premolars in dogs (From [21])

An accidental discovery during applying LIPUS to enhance bone formation at distraction site of the mandible in rabbits showed increased eruption of lower incisors with LIPUS compared to non-LIPUS-treated mandibles (El-Bialy et al., 2003). This discovery was further confirmed in an ex vivo mandible slice organ culture ([29], [Fig. 8.3]) and in animals ([21], [Fig. 8.4]). A multicenter, double-blinded, controlled clinical trial showed that LIPUS enhances rate of tooth movement during orthodontic treatment (unpublished data) (Fig. 8.5).

8.2   Orthodontics and Jaw Position Discrepancy

As mentioned above, orthodontic treatment involves correcting bad bites (malocclusion) that maybe created by jaw size–tooth size discrepancy or discrepancy between upper and lower jaw size/position.

When a discrepancy exists between upper and lower jaw sizes, malocclusion may occur if there is no dental compensation of the skeletal (jaw)

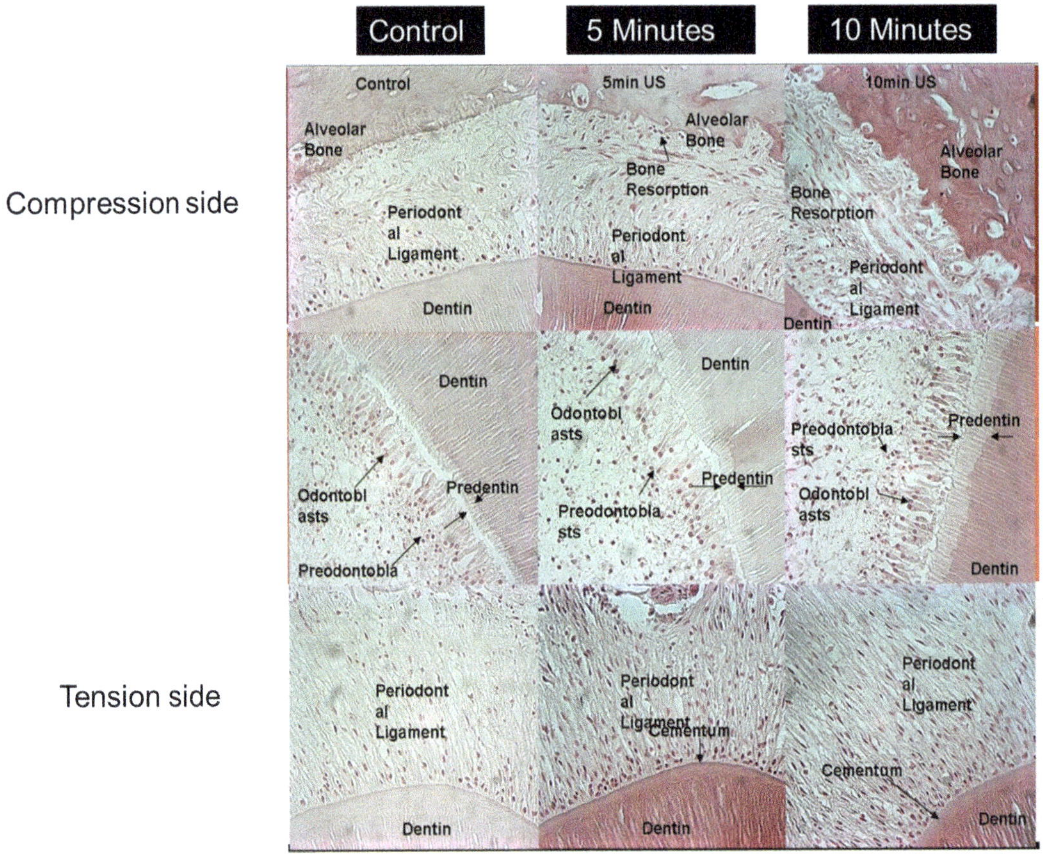

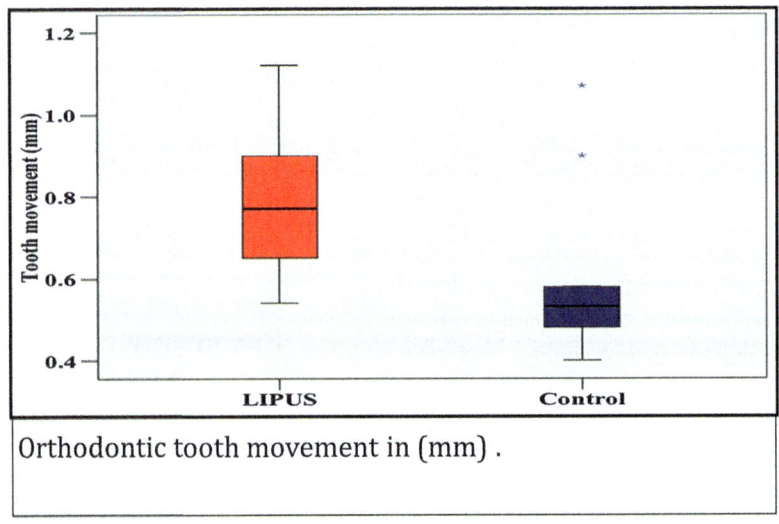

Fig. 8.3 In the ten minutes treated mandible slice organ culture at the compression side (top right corner), it can be noticed that there is increased alveolar bone remodeling with increased LIPUS compared to 5 min LIPUS-treated or control groups

Orthodontic tooth movement in (mm) .

Fig. 8.4 Rate of tooth movement in the LIPUS-treated and control premolars in beagle dogs [21]. It can be seen that LIPUS-treated premolars moved faster than control premolars over 28 days of daily LIPUS application to the experimental premolars in beagle dogs

Fig. 8.5 Left one of the compliant patients who had upper two first premolars removed for regular orthodontic treatment, you can notice that at the beginning (July 2014) extraction spaces were almost equal in size. After 4 months of space closure

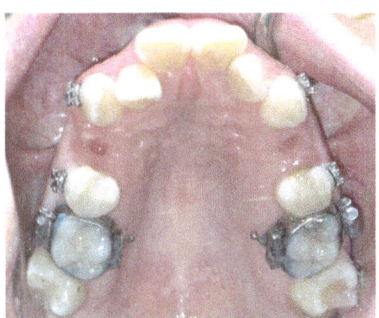 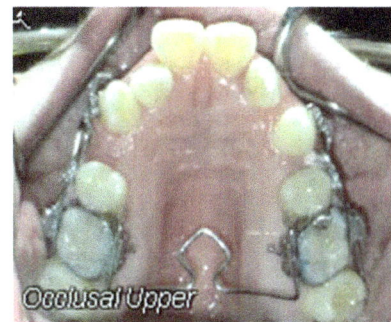

July 2nd 2014   Nov-5th, 2014

size discrepancy— an example of jaw size discrepancy in cases of normal size of the upper jaw and small or large size lower jaw or vice versa.

In the case of small sized lower jaw relative to a normal sized upper jaw, a malrelationship between the two jaws in the anteroposterior plane may exist; this is also known as skeletal class II relationship. This skeletal class II relationship may be also accompanied by dental arch malrelationship in the same way, which is also known as class II malocclusion. Although there are many varieties of class II malocclusion, it depends on the size and position of both upper and lower jaws relative to each other and relative to the cranial base, a commonly used skeletal reference in the craniofacial region. When the lower jaw is small in size and positioned backward relative to upper jaw, creating a class II skeletal and dental malocclusion, treatment options normally are directed to change the size and/or position of the lower jaw to a more forward position. Treatment modalities are mainly dependent on the age of the involved patient. In growing patients, treatment options normally involve what are called growth modification orthopedic devices or also known as functional appliances. Although these devices have been used widely in clinical orthodontics, the exact mechanism by which fictional appliances may change mandibular growth is still controversial and their effectiveness in modifying mandibular growth is still debatable in the literature.

This chapter presents the scientific evidence that low-intensity pulsed ultrasound (LIPUS) may be an adjunctive technique to functional appliances in order to enhance mandibular growth in cases with deficient or undergrown mandibles. Although a pilot study on the adjunctive use of LIPUS with functional appliances in cases with hemifacial microsomia has been published [25] (Fig. 8.6), the presented data suggested refinement of the techniques as it required daily application of LIPUS for an extended period of time between 6 and 12 months in order to observe clinical improvement in the patients' undergrown mandible sides. Although some attempts have been proposed in lower animals hypothesizing that increased daily LIPUS application (40 min) may enhance mandibular growth than 20 min daily application, current lower animal's results did not support this hypothesis [30]. One argument that could have led to the results that increased daily application of LIPUS from 20 to 40 min did not increase mandibular growth is that animals exposed to 40 min of daily LIPUS application were under more stress than those exposed to 20 min per day, as indicated by the decreased body weight of those animals treated by 40 min per day than those treated by 20 min LIPUS treatment. Further studies may be needed to confirm or otherwise refute this hypothesis.

In conclusion, the current literature supports that there is enough evidence that LIPUS application in orthodontics involves prevention of OIRR,

Fig. 8.6 A patient treated with hybrid functional appliance to allow for posterior teeth to grow on the right side and allows forward movement of the right side of the mandible to correct mandibular asymmetry to the patient's right side. LIPUS was applied to the patients' right side for twenty minutes per day for 8 months [25]

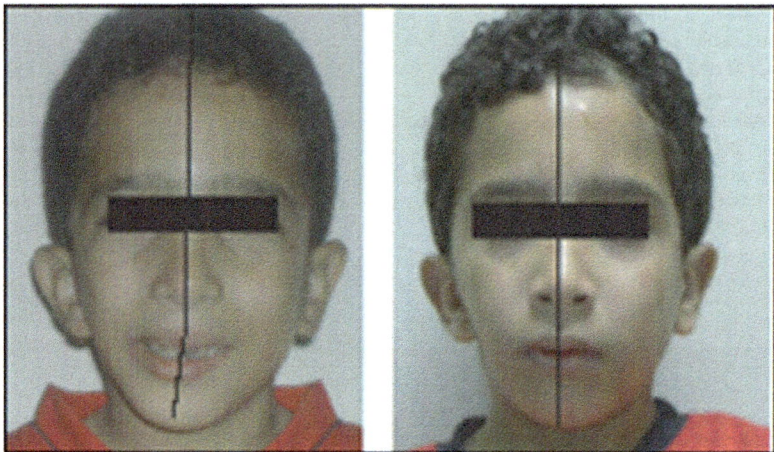

accelerates rate of tooth movement, as well as enhances mandibular growth in cases with under-developed mandibles and consequently can be an adjunctive treatment in class II malocclusion cases of skeletal origin.

References

1. Lupi JE, Handelman CS, Sadowsky C. Prevalence and severity of apical root resorption and alveolar bone loss in orthodontically treated adults. Am J Orthod Dentofacial Orthop. 1996;109:28–37.
2. Harris EF, Boggan BW, Wheeler DA. Apical root resorption in patients treated with comprehensive orthodontics. J Tenn Dent Assoc. 2001;81:30–3.
3. Mirabella AD, Artun J. Prevalence and severity of apical root resorption of maxillary anterior teeth in adult orthodontic patients. Eur J Orthod. 1995a;17:93–9.
4. Mirabella AD, Artun J. Risk factors for apical root resorption of maxillary anterior teeth in adult orthodontic patients. Am J Orthod Dentofacial Orthop. 1995b;108:48–55.
5. Linge BO, Linge L. Apical root resorption in upper anterior teeth. Eur J Orthod. 1983;5:173–83.
6. Killiany DM. Root resorption caused by orthodontic treatment: an evidence-based review of the literature. Semin Orthod. 1999;5:128–33.
7. Ishii M, Iwai K, Koike M, Ohshima S, Kudo-Tanaka E, Ishii T, et al. RANKL-induced expression of tetraspanin CD9 in lipid raft membrane microdomain is essential for cell fusion during osteoclastogenesis. J Bone Miner Res. 2006;21:965–76.
8. Vaananen K. Mechanism of osteoclast mediated bone resorption--rationale for the design of new therapeutics. Adv Drug Deliv Rev. 2005;57:959–71.
9. Sasaki T. Differentiation and functions of osteoclasts and odontoclasts in mineralized tissue resorption. Microsc Res Tech. 2003;61:483–95.
10. Low E, Zoellner H, Kharbanda OP, Darendeliler MA. Expression of mRNA for osteoprotegerin and receptor activator of nuclear factor kappa beta ligand (RANKL) during root resorption induced by the application of heavy orthodontic forces on rat molars. Am J Orthod Dentofacial Orthop. 2005;128:497–503.
11. Nakano Y, Yamaguchi M, Fujita S, Asano M, Saito K, Kasai K. Expressions of RANKL/RANK and M-CSF/c-fms in root resorption lacunae in rat molar by heavy orthodontic force. Eur J Orthod. 2011;33:335–43.
12. Seifi M, Jessri M. Expression of RANKL mRNA during root resorption induced by orthodontic tooth movement in rats. Yakhteh. 2009;11(3):293–8.
13. Yamaguchi M, Aihara N, Kojima T, Kasai K. RANKL increase in compressed periodontal ligament cells from root resorption. J Dent Res. 2006;85:751–6.
14. Harry MR, Sims MR. Root resorption in bicuspid intrusion. A scanning electron microscope study. Angle Orthod. 1982;52:235–58.
15. Owman-Moll P, Kurol J, Lundgren D. Repair of orthodontically induced root resorption in adolescents. Angle Orthod. 1995;65:403–8. discussion 409–410
16. Igarashi K, Adachi H, Mitani H, Shinoda H. Inhibitory effect of the topical administration of a bisphosphonate (risedronate) on root resorption incident to orthodontic tooth movement in rats. J Dent Res. 1996;75:1644–9.
17. Keum K-Y, Kwon O-T, ngberg LSS, Kim C-K, Kim J, Cho M-I, et al. Effect of dexamethasone on root resorption after delayed replantation of rat tooth. J Endod. 2003;29:810–3.
18. Aqrabawi J, Jamani K. Severe external root resorption arrested by conventional endodontic treatment. Dent Update. 2005;32:224–6.
19. El-Bialy T, El-Shamy I, Graber TM. Repair of orthodontically induced root resorption by ultrasound in

humans. Am J Orthod Dentofacial Orthop. 2004;126: 186–93.

20. Raza H, Major PW, Dederich D, El-Bialy T. Effect of low intensity pulsed ultrasound on orthodontically induced root resorption caused by torque: A prospective double blind controlled clinical trial. Angle Orthod. 2016 Feb;35(2):349–58.

21. Al-Daghreer S, Doschak MR, Sloane AJ, Major PW, Heo G, Scurtescu C, Tsui YY, El-Bialy T. Effect of LIPUS on orthodontically induced root resorption in Beagle dogs. Ultrasound Med Biol. 2014 Jun; 40(6):1187–96.

22. Inubushi T, Tanaka E, Rego EB, Ohtani J, Kawazoe A, Tanne K, Miyauchi M, Takata T. Low-intensity ultrasound stimulation inhibits resorption of the tooth root induced by experimental force application. Bone. 2013;53:497–506.

23. Liu Z, Xu J, E L WD. Ultrasound enhances the healing of orthodontically induced root resorption in rats. Angle Orthod. 2012;82:48–55.

24. Rego EB, Inubushi T, Miyauchi M, Kawazoe A, Tanaka E, Takata T, Tanne K. Ultrasound stimulation attenuates root resorption on rat replanted molars and impairs TNF-α signaling in vitro. J Periodont Res. 2011;46:648–54.

25. El-Bialy T, Hassan AH, Alyamani A, Albaghdadi T. Treatment of hemifacial microsomia by therapeutic ultrasound and hybrid functional appliance. A non-surgical approach. J Clin Trials. 2010;2:29–36.

26. Inubushi T, Tanaka E, Rego EB, Kitagawa M, Kawazoe A, Ohta A, Okada H, Koolstra JH, Miyauchi M, Takata T, Tanne K. Effects of ultrasound on the proliferation and differentiation of cementoblast lineage cells. J Periodontol. 2008;79: 1984–90.

27. El-Bialy TH, Zaki AE, Evans CA. Effect of ultrasound on rabbit mandibular incisor formation and eruption after mandibular osteodistraction. Am J Orthod Dentofac Orthop. 2003;124:427–34.

28. Rego EB, Inubushi T, Kawazoe A, Tanimoto K, Miyauchi M, Tanaka E, Takata T, Tanne K. Ultrasound stimulation induces PGE2 synthesis promoting cementoblastic differentiation through EP2/EP4 receptor pathway. Ultrasound Med Biol. 2010;36: 907–15.

29. El-Bialy TH, Lam B, Al-Daghreer SM, Sloan AJ. The effect of low intensity pulsed ultrasound in a 3D ex-vivo orthodontic model. J Dent. 2011;39: 693–9.

30. Kaur H, Uludag H, Dederich H, El-Bialy T. Dose dependent effect of low intensity pulsed ultrasound and bite jumping appliance on mandibular growth in rats. Ultrasound Med J. 2017;36(1): 109–20.

Clinical Application of LIPUS in the Dentofacial Region

Jacqueline Crossman, Harmanpreet Kaur, and Tarek El-Bialy

Abstract

The current scientific evidence supports that LIPUS has many clinical applications in the dentofacial region. This includes, but is not limited to, accelerating bone healing after any surgery, acceleration of soft tissue healing, accelerating tooth movement, and prevention of orthodontically induced root resorption. Also, there is strong evidence that LIPUS can be used in other dental applications like healing of dentoalveolar fractures after trauma. LIPUS also may help in dental pulp regeneration as well as periodontal regeneration. Moreover, LIPUS may aid in implant-bone integration. Details of these current and potential clinical applications are discussed.

The structures of the dentofacial region have unique development and function because they originate from neural crest and paraxial mesoderm [1]. These features limit the regenerative capacity of the tissues of the dentofacial region [1]. Oral and maxillofacial diseases, such as tooth decay, periodontal disease, dental pulp infection, and inflammatory root resorption, can seriously compromise the quality of life of millions of people worldwide [1]. To successfully re-create the compromised or missing dental tissues to their natural form would significantly and positively impact not only the lives of these affected patients but also the fields of dentistry, medicine, and tissue engineering, among many additional fields of research.

LIPUS has been proposed as an effective tool to enhance tissue engineering, which is generally limited by the scarceness of mesenchymal stem cell (MSC) numbers and the extended lab time required for growth and differentiation of the cells into target cells for incorporation into tissues [1]. LIPUS therapy is described as a "preferred bioreactor" [2] because it enhances angiogenesis [3–5], in addition to stimulating MSC growth and differentiation [6–8]. Increasing vasculature by LIPUS application is particularly important because vasculature is a requirement of integrating engineered tissue with native surrounding tissue.

In addition to in vivo studies demonstrating the therapeutic effects of LIPUS on promoting bone repair and regeneration, accelerating bone fracture healing, and enhancing osteogenesis at the distraction site, LIPUS has recently been reported to promote regeneration and

J. Crossman · H. Kaur
Department of Dentistry, University of Alberta, Edmonton, AB, Canada

T. El-Bialy (✉)
Dentistry/Orthodontics and Biomedical Engineering, University of Alberta, Edmonton, Alberta, Canada
e-mail: telbialy@ualberta.ca

healing in the dentofacial tissues. Al-Daghreer et al. [9] investigated the effect of LIPUS on the dentin–pulp complex using tooth organ slice culture (TOSC), an easy and reproducible in vitro model. A single application of LIPUS for 5 and 10 min significantly increased the expression of collagen I (Col I) and dentin matrix protein 1 (DMP1), respectively. Col I is the primary dentine matrix component [10]. DMP1 is an extracellular matrix protein associated with dentin mineralization and is present in dentin as well as in bone [11]. Since bone is not present in TOSC, the increased expression of DMP1 in this study is located within the dentin of the tooth slices. Research suggests that mesenchymal cell–DMP1 interactions at the extracellular level might be responsible for multiple signaling pathways that lead to ultimate differentiation into odontoblasts [12]. Furthermore, LIPUS increases odontoblast cell count and predentin thickness when applied for 5, 10 and 15 min [10]. Stimulating the secretion of extracellular matrix and associated protein in addition to increasing cellular layers, such as dentine, will improve resistance to bacterial or toxin penetration from cariogenic bacteria [10]. In addition, dentin layers that are denser may possibly be more resistant to dentin resorption [10]. This evidence and a recent clinical trial suggested that LIPUS can be used clinically in orthodontic patients with high risk of severe root resorption to prevent further orthodontically induced tooth root resorption [3, 13]. In addition, it has been demonstrated that LIPUS can also enhance tooth orthodontic movement in animals and in humans [3, 14]. This evidence can minimize other side effects of long orthodontic treatment. The effect of LIPUS on bone remodeling may be also a future technique that may be used to minimize relapse after orthodontic treatment. This, however, requires a long-term clinical trial to prove this possibility of clinical application.

Periodontal ligament cells (PDLCs) are the primary cellular component among the variety of other incorporated cell types in PDL tissues [15]. PDLCs maintain stem cell-like characteristics and can repair PDL tissues by synthesizing collagen and producing dental cementum [15]. Human PDLCs (HPDLCs) are considered a beneficial cell source for clinical periodontal regeneration [15]. The ability to stimulate HPDLC signaling pathways involved in early osteoblast differentiation, such as the mitogen-activated protein kinase (MAPK) signaling pathway, could accelerate soft-tissue healing [15]. HPDLCs exposed to LIPUS showed increases in alkaline phosphatase (ALP) activity and levels of osteocalcin, indicating early osteoblast differentiation of HPDLCs [15]. This study also reveals that the p38 MAPK signaling pathway is involved in this LIPUS-induced osteogenic differentiation [15]. Further research on the effect of LIPUS on PDL cellular function demonstrates that LIPUS can influence the production of key extracellular matrix proteins [16]. This study's variable findings emphasize the importance of determining and achieving optimal application parameters of LIPUS depending on the target cell population and tissue. Optimizing these parameters will continue to increase the understanding of the underlying mechanisms of how LIPUS can be used to repair and regenerate damaged tissues, such as PDL tissues.

LIPUS is being investigated for its potential application to accelerate postsurgical wound healing, such as recovery after gingival/periodontal flap surgery or dental implant surgery. LIPUS accelerates cementum and mandibular bone regeneration after flap surgery in the dog model, demonstrating that osteoblasts and PDL and gingival epithelium respond to LIPUS in increasing wound healing and bone repair [17]. LIPUS exposure further accelerates soft-tissue healing through connective tissue growth factor (CCN2/CTGF), which acts as a potent fibroblast mitogen and angiogenic factor and plays an important role in wound healing, regulation of extracellular matrix PDL tissue, cell proliferation, and angiogenesis [18]. This study further reported that the increase of CCN2/CTGF expression may be a result of the MAPK signaling pathway stimulated by LIPUS [18].

In addition to soft-tissue healing, further studies consider LIPUS's ability to repair hard tissue within the dentofacial region. The success rate of dental implants is relatively low for patients with either poor quantity or poor quality of alveolar bone. Furthermore, alleviating the inconvenience for patients by shortening rehabilitation time is an ever-increasing need [19]. Therefore, creating an easier, more effective method of osseointegration involved in dental implants is a necessity for dental clinicians and researchers. At a cellular level, LIPUS is effective at promoting proliferation and osteogenic differentiation of human alveolar bone-derived mesenchymal stem cells by positively influencing the expression of mRNA for ALP and Col I [19]. The underlying mechanisms involved in these cellular responses to LIPUS are still generally unknown; however, it has been demonstrated that LIPUS increases cyclooxygenase-2 (Cox-2) mRNA, which then leads to increased prostaglandin E2 (PGE2) [20]. These are proposed to play an essential role in the osseointegration of dental implants [21].

Beyond the cellular level of in vitro studies, LIPUS is effective in regenerating mandibular bone. Distraction osteogenesis has been considered a successful technique for gaining bone and soft-tissue mass in patients with a variety of craniofacial deformities [22]. In one study [23], rabbits underwent rapid mandibular osteodistraction and received LIPUS treatment for 1–4 weeks. After 4 weeks, regenerated bone completely filled the distraction gap with a thickened network of immature woven bone [22]. Osteoblasts predominantly characterized this region. Also, LIPUS significantly increased the bone volume/tissue volume percentage. The application of LIPUS in healing bone in maxillofacial fractures has also been proposed. Since the mandible is one of the most frequently involved bones in maxillofacial trauma, and a prolonged intermaxillary fixation period may result in temporomandibular joint disturbances, feeding impairment, and dental/periodontal problems because of difficulties in oral hygiene maintenance, evidence-based methods of accelerating mandibular fractures are necessary [23]. LIPUS has been shown to increase bone volume, trabecular thickness and separation, and bone density in mandibular fractures in the rabbit animal model [23]. This additional evidence demonstrates enhanced healing and bone formation by LIPUS treatment within the dentofacial

region. The clinical application of LIPUS after orthognathic surgeries including distraction osteogenesis is another feasible clinical application field.

Many studies provide research evidence of LIPUS's effect of increasing and enhancing tissue healing and regeneration within the dentofacial region. These studies include in vitro studies employing dentofacial cells and tissues and in vivo preclinical animal experiments. Additionally, a wide variety of results imply a range of the healing potential of LIPUS therapy. This is due to varying application parameters used within these studies. To further investigate LIPUS's potential of regenerating dentofacial tissues, and to move this field of research forward to more clinical trials, additional investigation must be emphasized on establishing the exact biological and biochemical mechanisms involved in LIPUS application and on determining optimal parameters of LIPUS stimulation required for particular tissue healing and regeneration.

Mandibular condylar growth stimulation in patients with deficient mandibles or patients with TMJ arthritis are other potential clinical applications of LIPUS. It has been shown that LIPUS enhances mandibular growth in rats, rabbits, and baboons and in human patients with hemifacial microsomia [24–27]. Also, it has been shown that LIPUS can enhance mandibular growth in arthritic mice [28, 29]. Future research needs to be conducted in order to verify the possible clinical application of LIPUS as an adjunct treatment in growing children with either undergrown mandibles and/or juvenile TMJ arthritis.

In conclusion, the current literature supports that LIPUS can be used clinically to minimize orthodontically induced tooth root resorption as well as to enhance orthodontic tooth movement. In addition, current literature supports the clinical application of LIPUS to enhance healing of bone and soft tissues after major surgeries. Also, current literature supports the possible application of LIPUS to enhance dental implant osseointegration and this would help in the future longevity of these implants. Future research still needs to be implemented to explore clinical efficacy of LIPUS in other dental clinical applications.

References

1. Tanaka E, Kuroda S, Horiuchi S, Tabata A, El-Bialy T. Low-intensity pulsed ultrasound in dentofacial tissue engineering. Ann Biomed Eng. 2015;43(4):871–86.
2. Nakamura T, Fujihara S, Katsura T, Yamamoto K, Inubushi T, Tanimoto K, Tanaka E. Low-intensity pulsed ultrasound reduces the inflammatory activity of synovitis. Ann Biomed Eng. 2011;39:2964–71.
3. Al-Daghreer S, Doschak M, Sloane A, Major P, Heo G, Scurtescu Y, Tsui Y, El-Bialy T. Effect of LIPUS on orthodontically induced root resorption in Beagle dogs. Ultrasound Med Biol. 2014;40:1187–96.
4. Dyson M, Pond J, Joseph J, Warwick R. The stimulation of tissue regeneration by means of ultrasound. Clin Sci. 1968;35:273–85.
5. Young S, Dyson M. The effect of therapeutic ultrasound on angiogenesis. Ultrasound Med Biol. 1990;16:261–9.
6. Angle S, Sena K, Sumner D, Virdi A. Osteogenic differentiation of rat bone marrow stromal cells by various intensities of low-intensity pulsed ultrasound. Ultrasonics. 2011;51:281–8.
7. Azuma Y, Ito M, Harada Y, Takagi H, Ohta T, Jingushi S. Low-intensity pulsed ultrasound accelerates rat femoral fracture healing by acting on the various cellular reactions in the fracture callus. J Bone Miner Res. 2001;16:671–80.
8. El-Bialy T, Alhadlaq A, Wong B, Kucharski C. Ultrasound effect on neural differentiation of gingival stem/progenitor cells. Ann Biomed Eng. 2014;42:1406–12.
9. Al-Daghreer S, Doschak M, Sloan A, Major P, Heo G, Scurtescu Y, Tsui Y, El-Bialy T. Short-term effect of low-intensity pulsed ultrasound on an ex vivo 3-d tooth culture. Ultrasound Med Biol. 2013;39:1066–74.
10. Al-Daghreer S, Doschak M, Sloan A, Major P, Heo G, Scurtescu Y, Tsui Y, El-Bialy T. Long term effect of low intensity pulsed ultrasound on a human tooth slice organ culture. Arch Oral Biol. 2012;57:760–8.
11. Balducci L, Ramachandran A, Hao J, Narayanan K, Evans C, George A. Biological markers for evaluation of root resorption. Arch Oral Biol. 2007;52(3):203–8.
12. Narayanan K, Srinivas R, Ramachandran A, Hao J, Quinn B, George A. Differentiation of embryonic mesenchymal cells to odontoblast-like cells by overexpression of dentin matrix protein 1. Proc Natl Acad Sci USA. 2001;98(8):4516–21.
13. Raza H, Major PW, Dederich D, El-Bialy T. Effect of low intensity pulsed ultrasound on orthodontically induced root resorption caused by torque: a prospective double blind controlled clinical trial. Angle Orthod. 2016;35(2):349–58.
14. El-Bialy T. Low intensity pulsed ultrasound accelerates tooth movement in human; 2017 Mar 25; IADR, San Francisco, Oral Presentation. ID#: 2626212.
15. Ren L, Yang Z, Song J, Wang Z, Deng F, Li W. Involvement of p38 MAPK pathway in low intensity pulsed ultrasound induced osteogenic differentiation of human periodontal ligament cells. Ultrasonics. 2013;53:686–90.
16. Harle J, Salih V, Mayia F, Knowles J, Olsen I. Effects of ultrasound on the growth and function of bone and periodontal ligament cells in vitro. Ultrasound Med Biol. 2001;27(4):579–86.
17. Ikai H, Tamura T, Watanabe T, Itou M, Sugaya A, Iwabuchi S, Mikuni-Takagaki Y, Deguchi S. Low-intensity pulsed ultrasound accelerates periodontal wound healing after flap surgery. J Periodontal Res. 2008;43:212–6.
18. Shiraishi R, Masaki C, Toshinaga A, Okinaga T, Nishihara T, Yamanaka N, Nakamoto T, Hosokawa R. The effects of low-intensity pulsed ultrasound exposure on gingival cells. 2011;82(10):1498-503.
19. Lim K, Kim J, Seonwoo H, Park S, Choung P, Chung J. In vitro effects of low-intensity pulsed ultrasound stimulation on the osteogenic differentiation of human alveolar bone-derived mesenchymal stem cells for tooth tissue engineering. Biomed Res Int. 2013;2013:1–15.
20. Kokubu T, Matsui N, Fujioka H, Tsunoda M, Mizuno K. Low intensity pulsed ultrasound exposure increases prostaglandin E2 production via the induction of cyclooxygenase-2 mRNA in mouse osteoblasts. Biochem Biophys Res Commun. 1999;256:284–7.
21. Chikazu D, Tomizuka K, Ogasawara T, Saijo H, Koizumi T, Mori Y, Yonehara Y, Susami T, Takato T. Cyclooxygenase-2 activity is essential for the osseointegration of dental implants. Int J Oral Maxillofac Surg. 2007;36:441–6.
22. El-Bialy T, Elgazzar R, Megahed E, Royston T. Effects of ultrasound modes on mandibular osteodistraction. J Dent Res. 2008;87(10):953–7.
23. Erdoğan Ö, Esen E, Üstün Y, Kürkçü M, Akova T, Gönlüşen G, Uysal H, Çevlik F. Effects of low-intensity pulsed ultrasound on healing of mandibular fractures: an experimental study in rabbits. J Oral Maxillofac Surg. 2006;64:180–8.
24. El-Bialy T, El-Shamy I, Graber TM. Growth modification of the rabbit mandible using therapeutic ultrasound: is it possible to enhance functional appliance results? Angle Orthod. 2003;73:631–9.
25. El-Bialy TH, Hassan A, Albaghdadi T, Fouad HA, Maimani AR. Growth modification of the mandible using ultrasound in baboons: a preliminary report. Am J Orthod Dentofac Orthop. 2006;130(10):435 e7–e14.
26. El-Bialy T, Hassan AH, Alyamani A, Albaghdadi T. Treatment of hemifacial microsomia by therapeutic ultrasound and hybrid functional appliance. A

non-surgical approach. Open Access J Clin Trials. 2010;2:29–36.

27. Oyonarte R, Zárate M, Rodriguez F. Low-intensity pulsed ultrasound stimulation of condylar growth in rats. Angle Orthod. 2009;79:964–70.

28. Alzaheri N, Abdallah MN, Crossman JJ, Tamimi F, Flood P, El-Bialy TH. Effect of ultrasound on condylar growth in juvenile arthritic mice; 2016 Jun; IADR Seoul, South Korea. Abstract ID #: 2474650.

29. Crossman J, Alzaheri N, Abdallah MN, Tamimi F, Flood P, El-Bialy T. Morphometric analysis of ultrasound-treated arthritic mouse model mandibles; 2017 Mar 23; IADR, San Francisco. Abstract #: 1288.

Clinical Application of Shockwave Therapy in Orthodontics

Dror Aizenbud and Hagai Hazan-Molina

Abstract

Extracorporeal shockwaves are noninvasive mechanical forms of sound wave treatment. They were introduced in medical therapy approximately 30 years ago in order to disintegrate kidney stones. Over the last 15 years, extracorporeal generated shockwaves have been used in many fields of medicine due to their versatility and ability to stimulate healing processes by inducing neovascularization and differentiate stem cells into cells of the injured tissue to allow proper healing and regeneration.

Orthodontic tooth movement is a model that includes the induction of aseptic inflammation and its resolution. Since extracorporeal shockwave therapy (ESWT) can modulate healing processes, it might have an effect on orthodontic tooth movement.

This hypothesis was recently studied in a rat model, in which rats were treated with ESWT in conjunction with orthodontic force commencement. After 3 days of force application, the concentration of all tested cytokines in the shockwave-treated group was smaller compared to the non-treated; however, a statistically significant difference was found only in regard to sRANKL. The anti-inflammatory effect and the positive effect of ESWT on bone formation are reflected in these results.

After 3 weeks of force application, the addition of ESWT to the orthodontic force further stimulated tooth movement by 45% when measured by microcomputed tomography. On the pressure side, the application of orthodontic force along with ESWT induced a significant decrease in volumetric bone mineral density, whereas orthodontic force alone did not. On the tension side, according to the accelerated tooth movement, a difference was observed in the newly formed bone between the groups.

These findings indicate that the induction of shockwave therapy during orthodontic tooth movement alternates the expression of different inflammatory cytokines in the PDL. This change might have been the cause of the increase in the rate of tooth movement by accelerating bone resorption on the pressure side and possibly enhancing bone formation on the tension side. Thus, ESWT might have a positive effect on bone turnover.

D. Aizenbud (✉) · H. Hazan-Molina
Technion—Faculty of Medicine, Oral Biology Research Laboratory, Rambam Health Care Campus, Haifa, Israel
e-mail: aizenbud@ortho.co.il

© Springer International Publishing AG, part of Springer Nature 2018
T. El-Bialy et al. (eds.), *Therapeutic Ultrasound in Dentistry*,
https://doi.org/10.1007/978-3-319-66323-4_10

10.1 Introduction

Extracorporeal shockwaves (ESW) are acoustic waves characterized by a lower frequency compared to other acoustic waves. Shockwaves can be exemplified in real life in daily phenomena such as a clapping sound, the sound of thunder following the flash of lightning, and the dramatic audible bang effect generated when an airplane breaks the sound barrier which can lead to the glass breaking even in distant areas. A shockwave is expected to be refracted, transmitted, or dissipated like any other waves entering live tissue. However, when clinically effective shockwaves enter the body, "controlled explosions" have been described [1]. According to the interfaces of different impedance values of the body structure, the shockwave energy will create compression and shear loads on the surface of the material with greater impedance. This rapid interaction between compression and shear forces results in cavitation. Microscopic gas bubbles are built up on the surface of the material with greater impedance, and the collapse of these bubbles creates a small jet of fast-flowing liquid that causes high local tension. This cavitation is believed to be responsible for the effects of ESW [2].

10.2 Shockwave: Physical Properties

Extracorporeal shockwaves (ESW) and low-intensity pulsed ultrasound (LIPUS) are non-invasive mechanical forms of sound wave treatment, with different magnitudes of stimuli [3]. ESW is clinically preferred because ESW requires fewer sessions, while LIPUS requires multitreatment settings for daily application over a period of time [4, 5].

When the speed of a source equals the speed of sound ($v = c$), the resulting wave forms a large amplitude, "sound barrier," as the wave fronts cannot escape the source. However, when the speed of a source exceeds the speed of sound ($v > c$), a cone-shaped "supersonic wave" front is formed with the source at the vertex. The wave fronts lag behind the source creating a large amplitude called a "shockwave." Unlike ordinary sound waves, the speed of a shockwave varies with its amplitude. The speed of a shockwave is greater than the speed of sound (Fig. 10.1). When a shockwave reaches an observer, a "sonic boom" is heard. Shockwaves die when their speed is reduced to an ordinary sound wave [6, 7].

A shockwave is defined as a sonic pulse characterized by an initial rapid rise in the positive pressure up to 100 megapascals (MPa) in less than 10 ns (nanoseconds) (1 MPa is about 10 times the atmospheric pressure = 1000 bar). The pressure will rapidly fall to a negative pressure of about 5–10 MPa reflected in a low tensile amplitude-relaxation phase (Fig. 10.2). The shockwaves build up very rapidly and have a short life cycle of approximately 10 microseconds and a broad frequency spectrum in the range of 16–20 MHz [8].

A metallic reflector in the shape of a half-ellipsoid focuses the almost spherical shock front, which is generated in the first focal point of the ellipsoid, to a second focal point.

Shockwaves can be generated from electrohydraulic, electromagnetic, or piezoelectric sources. In an electrohydraulic generator (used for bladder stone lithotripsy), an underwater electrode is discharged, which induces evaporation of water and causes a high-pressure wave. This is focused by an ellipsoidal reflector (which contains the first focal point) to generate a shockwave at the second focal point (the stone). This is the oldest principle of shockwave generation that produces high disintegrative capacity but also causes considerable pain.

Today, it is believed that the shockwave mechanisms are based on cellular and molecular actions which do not necessarily require focusing. Electromagnetic generators (that work in a way similar to loudspeakers) produce acoustic waves that are focused by means of a paraboloid reflector. The resulting shockwaves are almost parallel with a diameter the size of the reflector in order to apply the shockwaves to a larger area while reducing the number of shockwaves required to cover the predefined area, e.g., for wound therapy.

Fig. 10.1 The generation of a shockwave

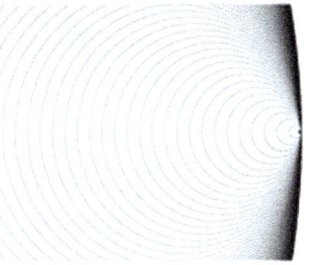
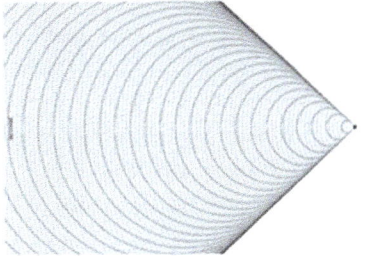

Source equals the speed of sound (*v* = *c*)

Wave fronts cannot escape the source

Speed of a source exceeds the speed of sound (*v* > *c*)

Wave fronts lag behind the source in a cone-shaped region with the source at the vertex

Fig. 10.2 The physical properties of a shock wave

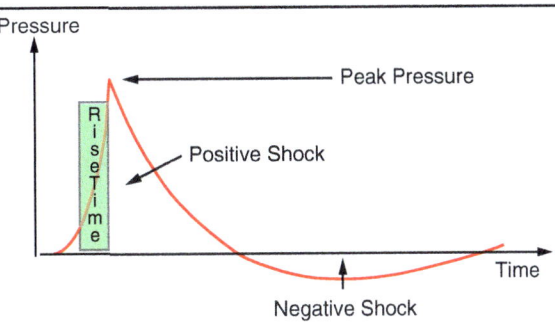

Profile of a typical shockwave: Pressure as a function of time of a shockwave. Rapid rise of positive peak pressure followed by a negative peak pressure6

Piezoelectric generators consist of multiple spherically aligned piezoelements, which induce high peak pressure in a small focal point. The resulting shockwave induces little pain. Consequently, these machines can be used without any need of sedation. The disadvantages of these generators are the large diameter of the source, the limited total energy in the focus, and the high re-treatment rate as a result of the low energy.

10.3 Shockwaves: The Biomechanical Effect on Tissue

Shockwave therapy in all of the medical fields serves as a stimulation of the healing processes by inducing neovascularization and differentiation of stem cells into cells of the injured tissue to allow proper healing and regeneration [9, 10]. This is a completely different approach compared to urology where shockwaves have been used for kidney stone disintegration.

Nitrogen oxide (NO) was hypothesized to play a dominant role in ESWT-mediated improvement of the blood flow. Increased nonenzymatic [11] and enzymatic (via upregulated nitric oxide synthase expression [12–14]) production of NO are discussed as possible scenarios for immediate improved tissue perfusion. In addition, the vascular endothelial growth factor (VEGF) increases in response to ESWT [14–18]. Furthermore, immunohistological studies evaluating vessel formation have demonstrated higher densities in the shockwave groups [9, 14, 17, 18]. Wang et al.

[19] showed Ras-dependent superoxide production following shockwave treatment which in turn regulates cytosolic ERK phosphorylation and HIF-1α transactivation. These intracellular changes may induce VEGF-A expression with subsequent angiogenesis.

Experimental studies on primary cultured human tenocytes demonstrated that ESWT enhances collagen synthesis and cell proliferation [20]. Furthermore, ESWT was reported to enhance the expression of transforming growth factor beta (TGF-β), which is proposed to be involved in chemotactic and mitogenic recruitment and differentiation of mesenchymal stem cells (MSCs) to cells of the injured tissue, thus assisting its regeneration [21, 22].

In addition, ESWT may have an anti-inflammatory mechanism. Early local inflammatory markers such as MIP-1α and MIP-1β were elevated in the sham- treated animals compared to ESWT-treated grafts, and the migration of leukocytes and macrophages was reduced significantly [12, 23]. Low energy shockwave therapy also efficiently downregulates nuclear factor κb (NF-κb) activation and NF-κb-dependent gene expression, thus diminishing pro-inflammatory stimuli [12, 23].

Locally (e.g., at the wound site) ESWT enhances cell proliferation [12, 24–26], stimulates extracellular matrix metabolism [24], decreases apoptosis [12, 27], and downregulates oxygen-regulated burst of leukocytes. Nonetheless, superoxide was found to promote shockwave-induced VEGF expression to a certain degree [19].

Moreover, ESWT may induce cell differentiation. Treatment of non-ischemic and chronic ischemic tissue with extracorporeal shockwaves has been found to be linked to improved homing of endothelial progenitor cell recruitment due to the limited presence of such factors [27]. In addition, stimulation of the bone marrow-derived mononuclear cells with shockwaves forces cell differentiation in an endothelial phenotype (VEGF[+], and CD31[+]) [28]. A similar effect was demonstrated in an in vivo segmental bony defect model but with osteoblastic differentiation [29]. ESWT produced maturation of human bone osteoblasts [25] and stimulated osteoblasts in cell cultures via increased release of alkaline phosphatase and osteocalcin [30].

10.4 Shockwaves Therapies: Application in Medicine and Dentistry

To date, ESWT has become increasingly popular and accepted worldwide. Successful application has been reported in numerous medical fields such as traumatology, veterinary medicine, treatment of impaired wound healing, burn injuries, and even erectile dysfunction. Indications for treatment with shockwaves were published at the 8th International Society for Medical Shockwave Treatment (ISMST) congress [31]. These indications include:

1. Chronic tendinopathies
2. Plantar fasciitis with or without heel spur
3. Radial epicondylopathy (tennis elbow)
4. Greater trochanteric pain syndrome
5. Delayed bone healing
6. Stress fractures
7. Early stage of avascular bone necrosis
8. Early stage of osteochondritis dissecans
9. Lithotripsy   (extracorporeal   and endocorporeal)
10. Muscular pathologies: Myofascial syndrome (fibromyalgia excluded) and injury without discontinuity.
11. Impaired wound healing
12. Burn injuries
13. Salivary stones

Despite this encouraging progress, the biomolecular basis by which shockwaves exert their positive effects is not yet completely understood. The advantages of extracorporeal shockwave therapy lay in its non-invasiveness (avoidance of surgery), low complication rates (e.g., petechial bleeding, hematoma), effectiveness in cases where there are indications of non-response to standard therapy, short learning curve, and its cost-effectiveness.

Shockwaves can be subdivided into energy categories based on the energy density that is generated by each machine [32]: low—< 0.08 mJ/mm^2, medium—0.08–0.28 mJ/mm^2, and high—>0.6 mJ/mm^2. Treatment protocol for shockwave therapy is dependent upon the energy category. With high-energy machines, such as machines used for bladder stone lithotripsy, the treatment course usually consists of 1000–4000 pulses for complete stone fragmentation [33]. In some cases, there might be a need for additional treatment. Usually high-energy therapy requires at least a local anesthetic and uses imaging technology to locate the treatment area. For low-energy machines, such as in the case of treatment of salivary calculi or different orthopedic pathologies, the treatment course consists of several treatments of 500–3000 pulses with the option of two to four additional treatments [34, 35]. Usually, no anesthesia is required for low-energy therapy. The treatment area is located by patient biofeedback on the area of greatest discomfort. Continuous sonographic monitoring allows direct visualization of the degree of fragmentation during treatment and avoids lesions to the surrounding tissues [36, 37]. Table 10.1 summarizes ESWT's characteristics in the different fields of medicine.

There is a great controversy with reference to the number of ESWT sessions required for a therapeutic effect. To date, no published data have evaluated whether there is a dose-dependent relationship between the outcome and the number of ESWT sessions the patient undergoes. Among the published cohort studies in the field of orthopedics, there does not seem to be a large difference in outcomes between studies that have used multiple and single sessions [34].

Several reports have described additional application of ESWT in the oral tissue. ESWT has demonstrated its potential in the removal of tooth biofilm [38] and its significant microbicidal effects on streptococcus mutans and an unencapsulated strain of *Porphyromonas gingivalis* following as few as 100 pulses at energy flux density (EFD) of 0.3 mJ/mm^2 ($p \leq 0.001$) [39]. These findings suggest that low-energy ESWT may be bactericidal for selected oral bacteria. Sathishkumar et al. [10] described the application of ESWT as an adjunct in the regeneration of periodontal tissues following *Porphyromonas gingivalis*-induced periodontitis. Infected rats treated with 300 and 1000 impulses demonstrated significantly improved alveolar bone levels at 3 weeks compared with untreated controls, and the improved levels remained for at least 6 weeks in most of the rats. In a sample of orthodontic patients, Falkensammer et al. found that ESWT had no statistically significant effect on pulpal blood flow [40]; nevertheless more rapid reduction in tooth mobility, probing depth, and bleeding on probing were achieved in the treatment group following treatment [41].

10.5 Shockwaves: The Rationale and Effect in Orthodontic Tooth Movement

Orthodontic tooth movement is achieved by the remodeling of periodontal ligament (PDL) and alveolar bone in response to mechanical loading [42, 43]. The transduction of mechanical forces to the cells triggers a biologic response, which has been described as an aseptic inflammation because it is mediated by a variety of inflammatory cytokines and does not represent a

Table 10.1 ESWT's characteristics in the different fields of medicine

Field of treatment	Energy category	Number of pulses	Number of appointments
Urology (bladder stone lithotripsy)	High	1000–4000	Usually 1
Salivary stone lithotripsy	Low	500–2000	2–4
Orthopedics (calcifying tendinitis, tennis elbow, heel spur, etc.)	Low	2000–3000	3–5
Erectile dysfunction problems	Low	300	2

pathological condition [44, 45]. In contrast to chronic inflammatory responses, in which persistent stimuli sustain a long-lasting inflammatory response and result in tissue damage, the expression of inflammatory mediators after orthodontic force application is transitory and essential for orthodontic movement, as anti-inflammatory drugs are capable of blocking tooth movement [46].

This tissue response initially involves vascular changes, followed by the synthesis of prostaglandins, cytokines, and growth factors. Finally, such mediators are believed to activate tissue remodeling, characterized by selective bone resorption or deposition in the compression and tension regions of the PDL, respectively [42, 43, 47]. Both soft and mineralized connective tissue metabolism can be modulated by cytokines and growth factors, pointing to the possible involvement of such factors in tissue remodeling during orthodontic tooth movement [48].

Rygh and Reitan [49] divided this biologic response into three phases of orthodontic tooth movement after the application of mechanical forces: initial tipping (several hours–~2 days after force application), lag phase (3–5 days after force application), and then tooth movement (7–14 days after force application). Rat models of tooth movement have provided in vivo evidence that IL-1β, TNF-α, and IL-6 are upregulated in PDL cells and osteoblasts [50, 51] and are important regulators in the bone remodeling process upon mechanical stimulation [52–54]. VEGF is the primary mediator of angiogenesis and serves various biological functions, such as increasing vascular permeability, promoting chemotaxis in human monocytes, and involvement in bone resorption and formation [55]. As a result, VEGF also plays an important role in orthodontic tooth movement [56]. All the cytokines are elevated in the gingival crevicular fluid of patients during orthodontic treatment within a few days after force application [54, 57, 58], i.e., during the tipping and lag phases.

Since ESWT can modulate healing processes, it might have an effect on orthodontic tooth movement.

The expressions and concentrations of IL-1β, IL-6, TNF-α, and sRANKL were evaluated in the gingival crevicular fluid and in the PDL and alveolar bone in rats after 3 days of orthodontic force application with/without ESWT [59, 60]. All cytokines displayed a similar trend in both the shockwave-treated and non-treated groups whereby the concentration peaked on the first day and declined thereafter. In all cases, the different cytokine concentrations in the shockwave-treated group were smaller compared to the non-treated; however, a statistical significant difference was found only in regard to sRANKL ($p = 0.011$) and a trend toward statistical significance was demonstrated in IL-6 on day 1 ($p = 0.065$). In the tissue, the percentage of cells expressing all inflammatory cytokines during the study's first two days was reduced in a statistically significant manner in the shockwave-treated group compared to the non-treated group. On the first day, the percentage of cells expressing IL-1β and RANKL in the compression side peaked in both groups, with a sequential rise in the number of tartrate-resistant acid phosphatase (TRAP)-positive cells. The anti-inflammatory effect and the positive effect of ESWT on bone formation are reflected in these results.

Moreover, recently, it was found that the addition of ESWT further stimulated tooth movement by 45% in the same rat model after 21 days of force application. Accordingly, a decrease in the volumetric bone mineral density (vBMD) and an increase in porosity (Po/Vo) were noticed on the pressure side in both groups, when measured by μCT; however, a greater decrease in vBMD was noticed in the rats that received ESWT in addition to the orthodontic appliance. Furthermore, a statistically significant increase in the number of TRAP-positive cells/area and in blood vessel density along with a greater expression of VEGF in the tissue were noticed in this group. All of the above indicate that a faster bone resorption occurs in the presence of ESWT, which is essential for accelerated orthodontic tooth movement.

The presence of immature, newly formed bone on the tension side was evidenced in the

Masson's trichrome stain and by the lower vBMD and greater PoV/TV and trabecular separation (Tb. Sp) in the group receiving ESWT in addition to the orthodontic appliance compared to the one that had only the orthodontic appliance, although the differences were not statistically significant. However, the difference between the groups became more evident when each group was compared to the control. On both the pressure and the tension sides, the additive effect of ESWT on orthodontic tooth movement was evident as the change in all microarchitectural parameters, measured in the μCT, was greater and statistically significant.

In light of the above, we can conclude that the application of shockwave therapy during orthodontic tooth movement increases the rate of tooth movement by accelerating bone resorption in the compression side and possibly enhancing the bone formation rate on the tension side. However, Falkensammer et al. [61] found no statistically significant differences in posterior–anterior tooth movement between the treatment and placebo group during the observation period in human subjects. The lack of difference could be for several different reasons. The ESWT protocol used was based on a protocol used in rats in previous reports [10, 59, 62, 63] and not in humans. In addition, the sample included non-growing patients, in whom Iwasaki et al. [64] observed a lower rate of tooth movement. Furthermore, multiple applications, i.e., a monthly application or higher energy flux densities of extracorporeal shockwaves, might show different effects. These could also be the reasons that Falkensammer et al. also did not find any differences in the pulpal blood flow in the same sample [40].

References

1. Ogden JA, Toth-Kischkat A, Schultheiss R. Principles of shock wave therapy. Clin Orthop Relat Res. 2001; 387:8–17.
2. Sturtevant B. Shock wave physics of lithotriptors. In: Smith A, Badlani G, Bagley D, editors. Smith's textbook of endourology. St. Louis, MO: Quality Medical Publishing; 1996. p. 529–52.
3. Li X, Chen M, Li L, Qing H, Zhu Z. Extracorporeal shock wave therapy: a potential adjuvant treatment for peri-implantitis. Med Hypotheses. 2010;74:120–2.
4. Qin L, Fok P, Lu H, Shi S, Leng Y, Leung K. Low intensity pulsed ultrasound increases the matrix hardness of the healing tissues at bone-tendon insertion-a partial patellectomy model in rabbits. Clin Biomech (Bristol, Avon). 2006;21:387–94.
5. Qin L, Wang L, Wong MW, Wen C, Wang G, Zhang G, et al. Osteogenesis induced by extracorporeal shockwave in treatment of delayed osteotendinous junction healing. J Orthop Res. 2010;28:70–6.
6. Elert G. The physics hypertextbook; 1998–2017.
7. Preminger GM. Shock wave physics. Am J Kidney Dis. 1991;17:431–5.
8. Vulpiani MC, Nusca SM, Vetrano M, Ovidi S, Baldini R, Piermattei C, et al. Extracorporeal shock wave therapy vs cryoultrasound therapy in the treatment of chronic lateral epicondylitis. One year follow up study. Muscles Ligaments Tendons J. 2015;5: 167–74.
9. Nishida T, Shimokawa H, Oi K, Tatewaki H, Uwatoku T, Abe K, et al. Extracorporeal cardiac shock wave therapy markedly ameliorates ischemia-induced myocardial dysfunction in pigs in vivo. Circulation. 2004;110:3055–61.
10. Sathishkumar S, Meka A, Dawson D, House N, Schaden W, Novak MJ, et al. Extracorporeal shock wave therapy induces alveolar bone regeneration. J Dent Res. 2008;87:687–91.
11. Gotte G, Amelio E, Russo S, Marlinghaus E, Musci G, Suzuki H. Short-time non-enzymatic nitric oxide synthesis from L-arginine and hydrogen peroxide induced by shock waves treatment. FEBS Lett. 2002;520: 153–5.
12. Kuo YR, Wang CT, Wang FS, Yang KD, Chiang YC, Wang CJ. Extracorporeal shock wave treatment modulates skin fibroblast recruitment and leukocyte infiltration for enhancing extended skin-flap survival. Wound Repair Regen. 2009;17:80–7.
13. Mariotto S, Cavalieri E, Amelio E, Ciampa AR, de Prati AC, Marlinghaus E, et al. Extracorporeal shock waves: from lithotripsy to anti-inflammatory action by NO production. Nitric Oxide. 2005;12:89–96.
14. Yan X, Zeng B, Chai Y, Luo C, Li X. Improvement of blood flow, expression of nitric oxide, and vascular endothelial growth factor by low-energy shockwave therapy in random-pattern skin flap model. Ann Plast Surg. 2008;61:646–53.
15. Kuo YR, Wu WS, Hsieh YL, Wang FS, Wang CT, Chiang YC, et al. Extracorporeal shock wave enhanced extended skin flap tissue survival via increase of topical blood perfusion and associated with suppression of tissue pro-inflammation. J Surg Res. 2007;143:385–92.
16. Ma HZ, Zeng BF, Li XL. Upregulation of VEGF in subchondral bone of necrotic femoral heads in rabbits with use of extracorporeal shock waves. Calcif Tissue Int. 2007;81:124–31.

17. Oi K, Fukumoto Y, Ito K, Uwatoku T, Abe K, Hizume T, et al. Extracorporeal shock wave therapy ameliorates hindlimb ischemia in rabbits. Tohoku J Exp Med. 2008;214:151–8.

18. Stojadinovic A, Elster EA, Anam K, Tadaki D, Amare M, Zins S, et al. Angiogenic response to extracorporeal shock wave treatment in murine skin isografts. Angiogenesis. 2008;11:369–80.

19. Wang FS, Wang CJ, Chen YJ, Chang PR, Huang YT, Sun YC, et al. Ras induction of superoxide activates ERK-dependent angiogenic transcription factor HIF-1alpha and VEGF-A expression in shock wave-stimulated osteoblasts. J Biol Chem. 2004;279: 10331–7.

20. Greve J, Grecco M, Santos-Silva P. Comparison of radial shockwaves and conventional physiotherapy for treating plantar fasciitis. Clinics (Sao Paulo). 2009;64:97–103.

21. Berta L, Fazzari A, Ficco AM, Enrica PM, Catalano MG, Frairia R. Extracorporeal shock waves enhance normal fibroblast proliferation in vitro and activate mRNA expression for TGF-beta 1 and for collagen types I and III. Acta Orthop. 2009;80:612–7.

22. Chen YJ, Wang CJ, Yang KD, Kuo YR, Huang HC, Huang YT, et al. Extracorporeal shock waves promote healing of collagenase-induced Achilles tendinitis and increase TGF-beta1 and IGF-I expression. J Orthop Res. 2004;22:854–61.

23. Davis TA, Stojadinovic A, Anam K, Amare M, Naik S, Peoples GE, et al. Extracorporeal shock wave therapy suppresses the early proinflammatory immune response to a severe cutaneous burn injury. Int Wound J. 2009;6:11–21.

24. Chao YH, Tsuang YH, Sun JS, Chen LT, Chiang YF, Wang CC, et al. Effects of shock waves on tenocyte proliferation and extracellular matrix metabolism. Ultrasound Med Biol. 2008;34:841–52.

25. Hofmann A, Ritz U, Hessmann MH, Alini M, Rommens PM, Rompe JD. Extracorporeal shock wave-mediated changes in proliferation, differentiation, and gene expression of human osteoblasts. J Trauma. 2008;65:1402–10.

26. Wang CJ. An overview of shock wave therapy in musculoskeletal disorders. Chang Gung Med J. 2003; 26:220–32.

27. Aicher A, Heeschen C, Sasaki K, Urbich C, Zeiher AM, Dimmeler S. Low-energy shock wave for enhancing recruitment of endothelial progenitor cells: a new modality to increase efficacy of cell therapy in chronic hind limb ischemia. Circulation. 2006;114: 2823–30.

28. Yip HK, Chang LT, Sun CK, Youssef AA, Sheu JJ, Wang CJ. Shock wave therapy applied to rat bone marrow-derived mononuclear cells enhances formation of cells stained positive for CD31 and vascular endothelial growth factor. Circ J. 2008;72:150–6.

29. Chen YJ, Wurtz T, Wang CJ, Kuo YR, Yang KD, Huang HC, et al. Recruitment of mesenchymal stem cells and expression of TGF-beta 1 and VEGF in the early stage of shock wave-promoted bone regeneration of segmental defect in rats. J Orthop Res. 2004;22: 526–34.

30. Martini L, Giavaresi G, Fini M, Torricelli P, de Pretto M, Schaden W, et al. Effect of extracorporeal shock wave therapy on osteoblastlike cells. Clin Orthop Relat Res. 2003;413:269–80.

31. Consensus statement. Recommendations for the use of extracorporeal shockwave technology in medical indications. 8th International congress of the ISMST Juan-les-Pins. 2008.

32. Rompe JD, Kirkpatrick CJ, Kullmer K, Schwitalle M, Krischek O. Dose-related effects of shock waves on rabbit tendo Achillis. A sonographic and histological study. J Bone Joint Surg Br. 1998;80:546–52.

33. D'Addessi A, Bongiovanni L, Sasso F, Gulino G, Falabella R, Bassi P. Extracorporeal shockwave lithotripsy in pediatrics. J Endourol. 2008;22:1–12.

34. Chung B, Wiley JP. Extracorporeal shockwave therapy: a review. Sports Med. 2002;32:851–65.

35. Nahlieli O, Shacham R, Zaguri A. Combined external lithotripsy and endoscopic techniques for advanced sialolithiasis cases. J Oral Maxillofac Surg. 2010;68: 347–53.

36. McGurk M, Escudier MP, Brown JE. Modern management of salivary calculi. Br J Surg. 2005;92: 107–12.

37. Ottaviani F, Capaccio P, Rivolta R, Cosmacini P, Pignataro L, Castagnone D. Salivary gland stones: US evaluation in shock wave lithotripsy. Radiology. 1997;204:437–41.

38. Muller P, Guggenheim B, Attin T, Marlinghaus E, Schmidlin PR. Potential of shock waves to remove calculus and biofilm. Clin Oral Investig. 2011;15: 959–65.

39. Novak KF, Govindaswami M, Ebersole JL, Schaden W, House N, Novak MJ. Effects of low-energy shock waves on oral bacteria. J Dent Res. 2008;87:928–31.

40. Falkensammer F, Schaden W, Krall C, Freudenthaler J, Bantleon HP. Effect of extracorporeal shockwave therapy (ESWT) on pulpal blood flow after orthodontic treatment: a randomized clinical trial. Clin Oral Investig. 2016;20:373–9.

41. Falkensammer F, Rausch-Fan X, Schaden W, Kivaranovic D, Freudenthaler J. Impact of extracorporeal shockwave therapy on tooth mobility in adult orthodontic patients: a randomized single-center placebo-controlled clinical trial. J Clin Periodontol. 2015;42:294–301.

42. Krishnan V, Davidovitch Z. Cellular, molecular, and tissue-level reactions to orthodontic force. Am J Orthod Dentofacial Orthop. 2006;129:469-e1.

43. Masella RS, Meister M. Current concepts in the biology of orthodontic tooth movement. Am J Orthod Dentofacial Orthop. 2006;129:458–68.

44. Meikle MC. The tissue, cellular, and molecular regulation of orthodontic tooth movement: 100 years after Carl Sandstedt. Eur J Orthod. 2006;28:221–40.

45. Wang XJ, Han G, Owens P, Siddiqui Y, Li AG. Role of TGF beta-mediated inflammation in cutaneous wound healing. J Investig Dermatol Symp Proc. 2006;11:112–7.
46. Walker JB, Buring SM. NSAID impairment of orthodontic tooth movement. Ann Pharmacother. 2001;35:113–5.
47. Cattaneo PM, Dalstra M, Melsen B. The finite element method: a tool to study orthodontic tooth movement. J Dent Res. 2005;84:428–33.
48. Kobayashi K, Takahashi N, Jimi E, Udagawa N, Takami M, Kotake S, et al. Tumor necrosis factor alpha stimulates osteoclast differentiation by a mechanism independent of the ODF/RANKL-RANK interaction. J Exp Med. 2000;191:275–86.
49. Rygh P, Reitan K. Ultrastructural changes in the periodontal ligament incident to orthodontic tooth movement. Trans Eur Orthod Soc. 1972;393–405.
50. Alhashimi N, Frithiof L, Brudvik P, Bakhiet M. Orthodontic tooth movement and de novo synthesis of proinflammatory cytokines. Am J Orthod Dentofacial Orthop. 2001;119:307–12.
51. Bletsa A, Berggreen E, Brudvik P. Interleukin-1alpha and tumor necrosis factor-alpha expression during the early phases of orthodontic tooth movement in rats. Eur J Oral Sci. 2006;114:423–9.
52. Le J, Vilcek J. Tumor necrosis factor and interleukin 1: cytokines with multiple overlapping biological activities. Lab Invest. 1987;56:234–48.
53. Ren Y, Hazemeijer H, de Haan B, Qu N, de Vos P. Cytokine profiles in crevicular fluid during orthodontic tooth movement of short and long durations. J Periodontol. 2007;78:453–8.
54. Uematsu S, Mogi M, Deguchi T. Interleukin (IL)-1 beta, IL-6, tumor necrosis factor-alpha, epidermal growth factor, and beta 2-microglobulin levels are elevated in gingival crevicular fluid during human orthodontic tooth movement. J Dent Res. 1996;75: 562–7.
55. Mayr-Wohlfart U, Waltenberger J, Hausser H, Kessler S, Gunther KP, Dehio C, et al. Vascular endothelial growth factor stimulates chemotactic migration of primary human osteoblasts. Bone. 2002;30:472–7.
56. Miyagawa A, Chiba M, Hayashi H, Igarashi K. Compressive force induces VEGF production in periodontal tissues. J Dent Res. 2009;88:752–6.
57. Grieve WG 3rd, Johnson GK, Moore RN, Reinhardt RA, DuBois LM. Prostaglandin E (PGE) and interleukin-1 beta (IL-1 beta) levels in gingival crevicular fluid during human orthodontic tooth movement. Am J Orthod Dentofacial Orthop. 1994;105: 369–74.
58. Lowney JJ, Norton LA, Shafer DM, Rossomando EF. Orthodontic forces increase tumor necrosis factor alpha in the human gingival sulcus. Am J Orthod Dentofacial Orthop. 1995;108:519–24.
59. Hazan-Molina H, Aizenbud I, Kaufman H, Teich S, Aizenbud D. The Influence of Shockwave Therapy on Orthodontic Tooth Movement Induced in the Rat. Adv Exp Med Biol. 2016;878:57–65.
60. Hazan-Molina H, Reznick AZ, Kaufman H, Aizenbud D. Periodontal cytokines profile under orthodontic force and extracorporeal shock wave stimuli in a rat model. J Periodontal Res. 2015;50:389–96.
61. Falkensammer F, Arnhart C, Krall C, Schaden W, Freudenthaler J, Bantleon HP. Impact of extracorporeal shock wave therapy (ESWT) on orthodontic tooth movement-a randomized clinical trial. Clin Oral Investig. 2014;18:2187–92.
62. Hazan-Molina H, Kaufman H, Reznick ZA, Aizenbud D. Orthodontic tooth movement under extracorporeal shock wave therapy: the characteristics of the inflammatory reaction--a preliminary study. Refuat Hapeh Vehashinayim. 2011;28:55–60, 71.
63. Hazan-Molina H, Reznick AZ, Kaufman H, Aizenbud D. Assessment of IL-1beta and VEGF concentration in a rat model during orthodontic tooth movement and extracorporeal shock wave therapy. Arch Oral Biol. 2013;58:142–50.
64. Iwasaki LR, Crouch LD, Tutor A, Gibson S, Hukmani N, Marx DB, et al. Tooth movement and cytokines in gingival crevicular fluid and whole blood in growing and adult subjects. Am J Orthod Dentofacial Orthop. 2005;128:483–91.

Pulp Cell Differentiation and Future Directions of LIPUS

11

Tarek El-Bialy

Abstract

Dental pulp tissue engineering has gone a long ways from proof of principle to clinical trials. However, the current clinical trials are limited to the utilization of the same patient's own dental pulp from another tooth to be removed and to be used to tissue engineer other teeth dental pulp. Dental pulp cell differentiation into different cell linages has been extensively investigated, although the potential use of LIPUS to enhance dental pulp cell differentiation still needs to be explored. This chapter will shed the light on the potential use of LIPUS in tissue engineering dental pulp regardless of the origin of stem cells used in tissue engineered dental pulp. According to the current literature, there is strong evidence that low-intensity pulsed ultrasound (LIPUS) can enhance the body regeneration process after trauma to most tissues. This accelerating regeneration process includes but not limited to many of the dentofacial tissues that have been tested so far except dental enamel. In orthodontics, LIPUS can minimize orthodontically induced teeth root resorption when it is applied during orthodontic treatment by stimulating new cementum and dentin formation that works as a protective layer against root resorption. Also, there is an adequate evidence that LIPUS can also enhance tooth movement at the same time. In addition, LIPUS can stimulate mandibular growth in growing animals and patients. Moreover, the stimulatory effect of LIPUS in enhancing the production of dental and other craniofacial tissue matrices plays an important role in regenerative dentistry, including but not limited to endodontics, dental traumatology, and jaw growth modification and maybe beyond these applications. This chapter also sheds light on these possible future applications as well.

11.1 Introduction

Recent reports have shown that dental pulp cells can be used for different organs tissue engineering as well as different tissue therapies. A recent report highlighted the techniques of isolating stem cells from dental tissues and their possible applications in dentofacial tissue engineering [1–4]. These applications include dentin [5], odontogenic and osteogenic differentiation [6], de novo living dental pulp [7], dental pulp regeneration [8], and recently neural differentiation [9]. The origin of these cells from neural crest and paraxial mesoderm makes them more

T. El-Bialy (✉)
Dentistry/Orthodontics and Biomedical Engineering, University of Alberta, Edmonton, Alberta, Canada
e-mail: telbialy@ualberta.ca

© Springer International Publishing AG, part of Springer Nature 2018
T. El-Bialy et al. (eds.), *Therapeutic Ultrasound in Dentistry*,
https://doi.org/10.1007/978-3-319-66323-4_11

attractive to be used for craniofacial tissue regeneration and tissue engineering [10, 11]. The scarcity of these cells and limited resources (limited to available dental pulp cells and or deciduous teeth) make the use of them not very practical should the receiver patient be edentulous or not have stored deciduous teeth to isolate these cells from them. Low-intensity pulsed ultrasound (LIPUS) has been reported to be an enhancer tool in tissue engineering, specifically when the mesenchymal stem cell (MSC) numbers are limited or scarce [11]. In addition, LIPUS therapy has been described as a "preferred bioreactor" [12] because it increases angiogenesis [13–15]. Moreover, it has been reported to stimulate MSC growth and differentiation [16–18]. In cases of limited dental pulp stem cells, LIPUS may be used as an adjunctive tool to enhance dental pulp stem cells' expansion and differentiation [19]. It has been reported that LIPUS enhances vascularity in dental pulp during tooth movement [13]. Moreover Al-Daghreer et al. [20, 21] and El-Bialy et al. [22] reported that LIPUS enhances sub-odontoblasts in human teeth slice organ culture and in rat mandible slice organ culture. The stimulatory effect of LIPUS to dental pulp stem cells suggests that LIPUS may be used in the dental pulp tissue engineering and/or regeneration.

Also, the stimulatory effect of LIPUS on sub-odontoblastic cell layer in slice organ culture as well as on odontoblasts in tissue culture [23] suggests that LIPUS may be used to regenerate dentin defects, for example, tooth fracture due to dental trauma [24]. A detailed prospective clinical trial is needed to test the feasibility of LIPUS to be an adjunctive treatment in repairing dentoalveolar fractures. A preliminary study has suggested that LIPUS can enhance neural differentiation of gingival cells which may be used for future dental pulp tissue engineering [18].

The propagation of LIPUS through dental tissue has been confirmed recently by Ghorayeb et al. [19] which suggests that LIPUS can effectively stimulate dental pulp cells when it is applied to the outside of teeth. The current literatures suggest different LIPUS outputs when considering applying LIPUS to dental tissues; however, the stimulatory effect may be different to different LIPUS outputs (frequency and intensities). Future research is needed to study different and optimum LIPUS parameters on different dental pulp cells (expansion and differentiation to different lineages).

Although it has not been investigated before, the current literature may suggest that LIPUS may be useful in the future to regenerate dentin in cases with severe dentinal defect like in large cavities due to dental caries. Also, preliminary results have shown that LIPUS can enhance tooth root length in amelogenin knockout mice [25]. In this type of mice it has been reported that amelogenin is vital to enamel growth and enamel crystal formation/growth [26]. Although our results on the effect of LIPUS on Amelogenine knockout mice are very preliminary, one might speculate or hypothesize that future research may prove that LIPUS may help in enamel formation and regeneration.

11.2 Summary of Dental Pulp Cell Stimulation by LIPUS

In conclusion, the current literature suggests that LIPUS has stimulatory effect on dental pulp cells as well as odontoblasts and cementoblasts. Collectively, it can be hypothesized that LIPUS can be used in the future for healing of dentoalveolar fractures and or root canal treatment.

11.3 Current Evidence of LIPUS Applications and Its Future Applications

The noninvasive behavior of LIPUS therapy is a promising tool for repair and regeneration of human tissues, including orofacial/dentofacial tissues with the exception of dental enamel as of now. LIPUS is currently widely employed in the medical field, such as orthopedic surgery and rehabilitation; however, its availability in other professional fields, such as dentistry, is still underutilized. LIPUS application to bony tissues is well investigated and has long been utilized in clinical orthopedics, but information is still lacking on its potential uses in dentofacial tissues, such as alveolar and mandibular bone, the TMJ, gingival and periodontal tissues, and the tooth and tooth roots with their associated tissues. Extensive research has being performed on understanding LIPUS's effects on healing tissues and the mechanisms by which these effects are present.

The mode by which LIPUS mechanically stimulates tissues is still unclear. However, it is known that LIPUS upregulates expression of bone formation-related genes, promotes protein synthesis and calcium uptake, and increases cellular differentiation [11]. Taken together, foundational knowledge is accumulating about LIPUS's mechanism and mechano-transduction, which can be used to build additional research upon to further the study of this field of regeneration research.

There is enough evidence that shock waves have a potentially great effect in orthodontics, in particular to minimize root resorption, and may enhance tooth movement. Detailed clinical trial is yet to be performed to show its efficacy in clinical orthodontics.

11.4 Future of LIPUS and Shock Waves in Dentofacial Regeneration and Tissue Engineering

Currently, many studies, both in vitro and in vivo, evaluating the effect of LIPUS on various tissues and cell types have reported a variety of results. This variation in results is primarily due to the fact that these studies used different LIPUS parameters, such as length of time of LIPUS exposure, average intensities, and frequencies. Since the response of tissues and cells can vary depending on these particular parameters, there is a need for studies that can determine the optimal LIPUS parameters for specific cell type or tissue. Optimal parameters of LIPUS application need to be determined for each tissue or organ in order to achieve optimum clinical effect of LIPUS. More studies with more evidence are needed to support validity, reliability, and replicability of the current

published studies. Next, further biological and biochemical mechanisms of LIPUS effect need to be investigated. In order to perform these studies, close collaboration is needed between clinicians, basic scientists, and engineers.

There are ample of potential applications of LIPUS in dentofacial regeneration and tissue engineering. These applications can include, but not limited to the following applications:

1. Endodontics: The current evidence supports that LIPUS can differentiate undifferentiated cells from the gum into nerve-like cells. Also, there is strong evidence that LIPUS enhances vascularization, differentiates pre-odotoblasts into odontoblasts, and increases dentin formation. This evidence supports the hypothesis that LIPUS can be an adjunct tool to tissue engineer dental pulp or regenerate dental pulp after injury.

2. Dental trauma: There is substantial evidence that LIPUS enhances dental tissue formation including osteodentin (reparative dentin), cementum and dentin matrices, vascularity, and bone healing. The regeneration of these tissues is needed after dental trauma that may involve fractured tooth/teeth and alveolar bone; either the trauma may lead to devitalization of the involved tooth/teeth or not.

3. Oral surgery: After any surgical intervention, LIPUS can enhance healing of the affected tissues including bone, soft tissue, and/or dental tissue healing. Also, the possibility of using LIPUS to enhance matrix formation can be an excellent adjunct in tissue engineering of lost tissues like after major resection after trauma or tumors. Also, LIPUS may be helpful in cases with TMJ arthritis that currently may require extensive TMJ resection and/or replacement.

4. Prosthodontics: The possibility of tissue engineering teeth is not too far from reality. Tissue engineering requires plenty of cells and a technique that can help differentiate these cells into the proposed tissue cells as well as enhancing producing matrices of the differentiated cells. In addition, integration of the engineered tissue with the patient's organ requires an

enhancer that can help this integration. The current literature suggests that LIPUS can provide this role due to its reported lab and clinical application, acceptable performance, and safety.

5. Orthodontics: The current literature supports that LIPUS can prevent/minimize orthodontically induced tooth root resorption, accelerate orthodontic tooth movement, as well as stimulate mandibular growth, which are all challenges in current orthodontic practice.

6. Periodontics: There is strong evidence that LIPUS can regenerate alveolar bone and cementum after periodontal defects. Although the current evidence is limited to animal experiments, clinical application/trials are needed to prove or to optimize LIPUS application in periodontal regeneration.

7. Future exploration of the possible stimulatory effects of LIPUS on ameloblasts (the enamel forming cells) may be performed. Should scientific evidence prove that LIPUS can stimulate enamel matrix formation, future applications of LIPUS toward strengthening enamel formation during permanent tooth formation and eruption might be the future way of minimizing dental caries. The problem is still challenging after almost two centuries of scientific efforts that aimed at understanding and possibly minimizing dental caries.

8. Shock wave seems to be promising in minimizing root resorption and may enhance orthodontic tooth movement. Clinical trials are yet to be performed to prove this hypothesis or otherwise show different responses.

11.5 Summary

The current evidence supports that the future of LIPUS application in dentistry and dentofacial orthopedics/regeneration is huge and is expected to be in almost all dentistry fields. Having said this, there is a long road still ahead for these goals to be achieved. Extensive collaboration between different disciplines as well as different institutes

is needed in order to make these hypotheses a reality. Also, the new generation of researchers may be interested in continuing this research in there careers.

References

1. Huang GT, Gronthos S, Shi S. Mesenchymal stem cells derived from dental tissues vs. those from other sources: their biology and role in regenerative medicine. J Dent Res. 2009;88(9):792–806.
2. Sloan AJ, Smith AJ. Stem cells and the dental pulp: potential roles in dentine regeneration and repair. Oral Dis. 2007;13(2):151–7.
3. Souron JB, Petiet A, Decup F, Tran XV, Lesieur J, Poliard A, Le Guludec D, Letourneur D, Chaussain C, Rouzet F, Opsahl Vital S. Pulp cell tracking by radionuclide imaging for dental tissue engineering. Tissue Eng Part C Methods. 2014;20(3):188–97.
4. Duailibi MT, Duailibi SE, Duailibi Neto EF, Negreiros RM, Jorge WA, Ferreira LM, Vacanti JP, Yelick PC. Tooth tissue engineering: optimal dental stem cell harvest based on tooth development. Artif Organs. 2011;35(7):E129–35.
5. Zheng Y, Wang XY, Wang YM, Liu XY, Zhang CM, Hou BX, Wang SL. Dentin regeneration using deciduous pulp stem/progenitor cells. J Dent Res. 2012;91 (7):676–82.
6. Zou T, Dissanayaka WL, Jiang S, Wang S, Heng BC, Huang X, Zhang C. Semaphorin 4D enhances angiogenic potential and suppresses osteo-/odontogenic differentiation of human dental pulp stem cells. J Endod. 2017;43(2):297–305.
7. Bhoj M, Zhang C, Green DW. A first step in De Novo synthesis of a living pulp tissue replacement using dental pulp MSCs and tissue growth factors encapsulated within a bioinspired alginate hydrogel. J Endod. 2015;41(7):1100–7.
8. Dissanayaka WL, Hargreaves KM, Jin L, Samaranayake LP, Zhang C. The interplay of dental pulp stem cells and endothelial cells in an injectable peptide hydrogel on angiogenesis and pulp regeneration in vivo. Tissue Eng Part A. 2015;21(3-4):550–63.
9. Heng BC, Lim LW, Wu W, Zhang C. An overview of protocols for the neural induction of dental and oral stem cells in vitro. Tissue Eng Part B Rev. 2016;22 (3):220–50.
10. La Noce M, Mele L, Tirino V, Paino F, De Rosa A, Naddeo P, Papagerakis P, Papaccio G, Desiderio V. Neural crest stem cell population in craniomaxillofacial development and tissue repair. Eur Cell Mater. 2014;28(28):348–57.
11. Tanaka E, Kuroda S, Horiuchi S, Tabata A, El-Bialy T. Low-intensity pulsed ultrasound in dentofacial tissue engineering. Ann Biomed Eng. 2015;43(4):871–86.
12. Nakamura T, Fujihara S, Katsura T, Yamamoto K, Inubushi T, Tanimoto K, Tanaka E. Low-intensity

pulsed ultrasound reduces the inflammatory activity of synovitis. Ann Biomed Eng. 2011;39:2964–71.

13. Al-Daghreer S, Doschak M, Sloane A, Major P, Heo G, Scurtescu Y, Tsui Y, El-Bialy T. Effect of LIPUS on orthodontically induced root resorption in Beagle dogs. Ultrasound Med Biol. 2014;40:1187–96.

14. Dyson M, Pond J, Joseph J, Warwick R. The stimulation of tissue regeneration by means of ultrasound. Clin Sci. 1968;35:273–85.

15. Young SR, Dyson M. Effect of therapeutic ultrasound on the healing of full-thickness excised skin lesions. Ultrasonics. 1990;28(3):175–80.

16. Angle S, Sena K, Sumner D, Virdi A. Osteogenic differentiation of rat bone marrow stromal cells by various intensities of low-intensity pulsed ultrasound. Ultrasonics. 2011;51:281–8.

17. Azuma Y, Ito M, Harada Y, Takagi H, Ohta T, Jingushi S. Low-intensity pulsed ultrasound accelerates rat femoral fracture healing by acting on the various cellular reactions in the fracture callus. J Bone Miner Res. 2001;16:671–80.

18. El-Bialy T, Alhadlaq A, Wong B, Kucharski C. Ultrasound effect on neural differentiation of gingival stem/progenitor cells. Ann Biomed Eng. 2014;42(7):1406–12.

19. Ghorayeb SR, Patel US, Walmsley AD, Scheven BA. Biophysical characterization of low-frequency ultrasound interaction with dental pulp stem cells. J Ther Ultrasound. 2013;1(1):12.

20. Al-Daghreer S, Doschak M, Sloan A, Major P, Heo G, Scurtescu Y, Tsui Y, El-Bialy T. Long term effect of low intensity pulsed ultrasound on a human tooth slice organ culture. Arch Oral Biol. 2012;57:760–8.

21. Al-Daghreer S, Doschak M, Sloan A, Major P, Heo G, Scurtescu Y, Tsui Y, El-Bialy T. Short-term effect of low-intensity pulsed ultrasound on an ex vivo 3-d tooth culture. Ultrasound Med Biol. 2013;39:1066–74.

22. El-Bialy TH, Lam B, Al-Daghreer SM, Sloan AJ. The effect of low intensity pulsed ultrasound in a 3D ex-vivo orthodontic model. J Dent. 2011;39:693–9.

23. Scheven BA, Shelton RM, Cooper PR, Walmsley AD, Smith AJ. Therapeutic ultrasound for dental tissue repair. Med Hypotheses. 2009;73(4):591–3.

24. Law AG, Sadeghi H, Sloan A, El-Bialy T. Effect of low intensity pulsed ultrasound on dentoalveolar fracture in mandible slice organ culture; 2011 Mar; IADR, San Diego. Poster # 2907.

25. Alzaheri N, Nour M, Tamimi F, El-Bialy T. Low-intensity pulsed ultrasound increases teeth root volume in amelogenin knockout mice. Oral presentation. 2016 AADR/CADR Annual Meeting; 2016 Mar 18; Los Angeles, CA. ID#: 2399910.

26. Wright JT, Li Y, Suggs C, Kuehl MA, Kulkarni AB, Gibson CW. The role of amelogenin during enamel-crystallite growth and organization in vivo. Eur J Oral Sci. 2011;119(Suppl 1):65–9.

Index

The manufacturer's authorised representative in the EU is Springer
Nature Customer Service Centre GmbH, Europaplatz 3, 69115 Heidelberg,
Germany. If you have any concerns regarding our products, please
contact ProductSafety@springernature.com

Printed and bound by CPI Group (UK) Ltd, Croydon, CR0 4YY

24/04/2026

02096361-0001